The Romance of Remedies

A physician looks back

O . L . WADE

With a Foreword by
Professor Sir Michael Drury, O.B.E., F.R.C.P., F.R.C.G.P.,
F.R.A.C.G.P., Emeritus Professor of General Practice,
University of Birmingham.
One time President of the Royal College of General Practitioners.

Durham Academic Press

First published in 1996 by
Durham Academic Press
1 Hutton Close,
South Church
Bishop Auckland
Durham

ISBN 1-900838-02-8

Typeset by Carnegie Publishing, 18 Maynard St, Preston
Printed and bound by Antony Rowe Ltd, Chippenham

The Romance of Remedies

Contents

Illustrations

Foreword

I t is a salutary thought that anyone born after the
start of the Second World War has lived during the
period of discovery of virtually all the drugs in medical
use today. Indeed only a handful of drugs which were
used when I qualified in 1949 are now in common use.
As Professor Wade writes 'the excitement of discovering
something of help to patients is enormous' and the
excitement for the physician in having such discoveries
made available is no less great.

At times there seems to be a plethora of drugs and
currently there are more than 1800 available to each
general practitioner from which he regularly uses about
300. Each person in the population of this country
receives on average ten prescription items per year. Of
course it is true that some are not really necessary and
others are given to relieve the symptoms rather than
alter the nature of an illness, but that number still
contains many that cure or prevent life-threatening
disease and yet others that ease the burden of otherwise
intolerable illness.

What a remarkable story of endeavour and achieve-
ment this has been, the flavour of which is so beautifully
captured in this small book. There are several reasons
why this book should have been written but there is

probably only one person who could have captured the events in such a personal way. It is a tale told by one who not only lived through much of the time and witnessed it but whose work kept touching and retouching the subjects while they developed. To tell the story of just eight of these many drugs, even though they are eight of the most significant, may seem to do scant justice to the importance of the topic but if they are considered to be exemplars of the great pharmacological revolution the reader will be well served whether he or she approaches from a medical or other background.

The subject of medicines and their use and abuse have become part of the daily diet of every reader, listener or viewer. Rightly, patients now approach their drugs with more circumspection than they were wont to do. But it is too easy when considering the potential risks of treatment in a litigious age to forget the benefits. 'If you don't like the medicine try the disease' is the sort of remark that Mark Twain might have made and something all of us should remember. These pages will help to restore the balance.

Those of us who were privileged to watch and contribute to Professor Wade's teaching, research and patient care recognise the great contribution he made to understanding the proper place of medicines in patient care. This book should widen that appreciation.

Michael Drury
25 November 1995

Introduction

This book is a result of retirement, memories and a word processor. I am a physician and was a professor of therapeutics for thirty years. When I retired and was cut off from my patients and my clinical work I decided that I would do all the things I had always wanted to do but had been too busy to do when I was working.

In fact the transition from work to retirement was much more precipitate than I had expected. I had always thought that I would be able to spend the last year of my professional life tidying up my affairs and slowing down a bit. As it was I found myself by a cruel turn of events doing three jobs at once; I was Head of the Department of Therapeutics, Head of the Department of Medicine and Vice-Principal of the University of Birmingham.

I remember very vividly the first day of my retirement, 1 October 1986. It was an extraordinary delight to have a prolonged breakfast with Margaret and then to be able to read the newspaper in leisure. I only realised what a large burden work I had been carrying when I was relieved of it.

So Margaret and I felt young again. We did a lot of sailing. I did a lot of woodwork. Amongst other things

I made a settle, a chest of drawers, a dining table and a desk. I taught myself wood turning. I saturated my family with furniture and bowls. I did very little professional work; just a few tribunals and some work for the World Health Organisation which kept me in touch with old friends. Margaret was very active with her watercolours and with very original and creative embroidery.

My youngest daughter, Sian, is a nursing sister. I used to go round to her house and play with her word processor. My typing had never been very good but I and her word processor became very friendly. Very soon I found I needed to have one of my own and then I decided to write an autobiography for my grandchildren. I found this a very satisfying experience. I re-lived my life and I remembered much that I had long forgotten. And while doing this I looked again at old files which were full of my lecture notes, usually pretty scrappy but the headings brought back ideas and memories. And there were many memos and cuttings, for when I was working I was always making notes or was busy with scissors cutting out articles on subjects that interested me and stuffing them into my files. And suddenly I had an urge to write about some of the things that I had learnt concerning drugs which I had never had time to pass on to my students.

So this is what this book is about. I have picked on a few drugs the history of which I have found exciting or for which, for one reason or another I have had interesting, or to me memorable, associations. I hope

Introduction

that my readers will be as fascinated as I have been at these memories, some of which, I if I do not record them, will be lost for ever.

CHAPTER I

Quinine

The Fever Bark

The history of quinine is rich in religious controversy, political intrigue and commercial skulduggery. This is not surprising as it was the first, and for many years the only, effective treatment of fever caused by the malaria parasite. Even now, despite the development of effective synthetic antimalarial drugs, it is still an important therapeutic drug although far the greatest proportion of quinine that is now produced, is marketed commercially to the soft drinks industry to make tonic water.

The introduction of the bark to Europe

Long before anyone knew the cause of malaria the Spanish conquistadores in South America learnt that the natives had a remedy for 'fever'. In 1633 an Augustinian monk, Fr Calancha, wrote about the 'fever tree' of Loxa in Peru, the bark of which was used by the Indians to treat fever, and it was this bark which was used to treat with success the Viceroy of Peru, Don

Luis Geronimo Cabrera de Bobadilla, 4th Count of Chinchon. His wife, Condessa Anna del Chinchon, was also treated with the bark by her physician, Juan del Vego, who was deeply impressed at the speed of her recovery. At any rate, the tree from which the bark was obtained was later named the cinchona tree after the Viceroy by the great botanist Linnaeus, while the powdered bark which was first brought to Europe in 1639 or 1640 became known as the *polvo de la Condesa*.

It is likely that the Jesuit fathers were, at the beginning, the chief importers and distributors of the bark in Europe and its reputation as a remedy for 'fever' spread rapidly. Some who received the remedy had malaria which responded to it, but no doubt there were many who recovered from illnesses which were totally unrelated to malaria, and who then ascribed their recovery to the use of the 'the Jesuits' bark'.

Claims and counter claims

The aged Jesuit, Cardinal de Lugo, who taught at the Gregoria University in Rome, impressed by accounts of the effectiveness of the drug, instituted an inquiry into the properties of the bark by the Pope's physician, Dr Fonseca, and in 1651 had an account of its virtues published in a small booklet, the *Schedula Romana*.

However the remedy failed to cure the Archduke Leopold of Austria of a fever that he suffered and he ordered his physician, Joan Jacob Chiflet, to denounce the bark as a fraud. Chiflet did this in 1653 in a pamphlet entitled *Exposure of the Febrifuge Powder from the American World.* The Cardinal responded promptly and *A Vindication of the Peruvian Powder* was written on his behalf by Antimus Conyguis in the same year.

The Archduke Leopold regarded this as a personal insult and commissioned Professor Plumbous of Louvain to deal with the matter. This the Professor did in 1655 with considerable zest for he was a Jansenite believing in predestination and abhorring the Jesuits who believed in free will. He poured scorn on 'the powder of the most eminent Cardinal de Lugo'.

Eight years later Dr Sturm of Delft confirmed de Lugo's conviction that the bark was a valuable remedy, but by then the old Cardinal had died.

The introduction of the bark in England

Much of the credit for the introduction of the remedy to England must go to Robert Talbor. At a time when most physicians gave very large doses of the powder, which must have caused unpleasant symptoms of ringing in the ears, tinnitus, nausea and blurred vision, he used a regimen of small but frequent doses. He acquired a considerable reputation and in 1668 he moved from Essex to London and established himself as a 'pyretiatro' or fever doctor. In 1672 he published a book with the delightful title *Pyretologia, a Rational Account of the Cause and Cure of Agues: whereunto is added a short Account of the Cause and Cure of Feavers.*

Talbor soon had an enormous practice in London and in 1678 he treated Charles II so successfully that he was appointed a Physician to the King and knighted. The Secretary of State was commanded by the King to write to the Royal College of Physicians of London, which had regarded Talbor with disfavour thinking him a quack, to revise its opinion and recognise his competence.

In 1678 Charles commended Sir Robert Talbor to Louis XIV in Paris and the amazing cure of a fever which his son the Dauphin suffered, which was attributed to Talbor's intervention, had Madame de Sévigné in rapture about *le remède de l'anglais*. Louis brought the secret of the remedy from Talbor for 3000 crowns and a life pension. He created him Chevalier Talbot (note the change in name) and in 1682 had published a pamphlet, understandably translated into English immediately, on *The English Remedy or Talbor's Wonderful Secret for Curing of Agues and Feavers*. It was of course the Jesuit's powder in slight disguise.

There is a monument in Trinity Church, Cambridge with the following fulsome inscription to the memory of the:

most honourable Robert Talbor, Knight and singular physician, unique in curing fever of which he delivered Charles II, King of England, Louis XIV, King of France, the most serene Dauphine, princes, many a duke and a large number of lesser personages.

It is a comment on the ineffectiveness of many of the remedies which were in use in those times that Bernadino Ramazzini the Italian physician, who was a contemporary of Talbor, spoke of the introduction of the bark to European medicine as comparable in its effect to the introduction of gunpowder to the art of war. Ramazzini was an ardent supporter of the use of the bark for the treatment of 'intermittent' fevers but was, interestingly, much against its indiscriminate use in fevers which were not intermittent, and, of course, we now know the fever caused by malaria parasites is characteristically intermittent

It was many years later that Sir George Baker of the Royal College of Physicians of London gave to Sir Robert Talbor the credit for introducing and using the bark effectively in England.

The difficult and dangerous search for the source of the bark

Although by the beginning of the eighteenth century the South American bark was widely known and used in Europe, knowledge of its source was very limited and no doubt its supply was capricious for the Spanish colonists of New Granada, a territory which included modern Ecuador and Colombia, were far more interested in their trade in silver and slaves than in cinchona bark. See Fig. 1. 1

In 1735 a French geological expedition was sent to Ecuador to make measurements of the circumference of the earth. One of the members was the scientist De

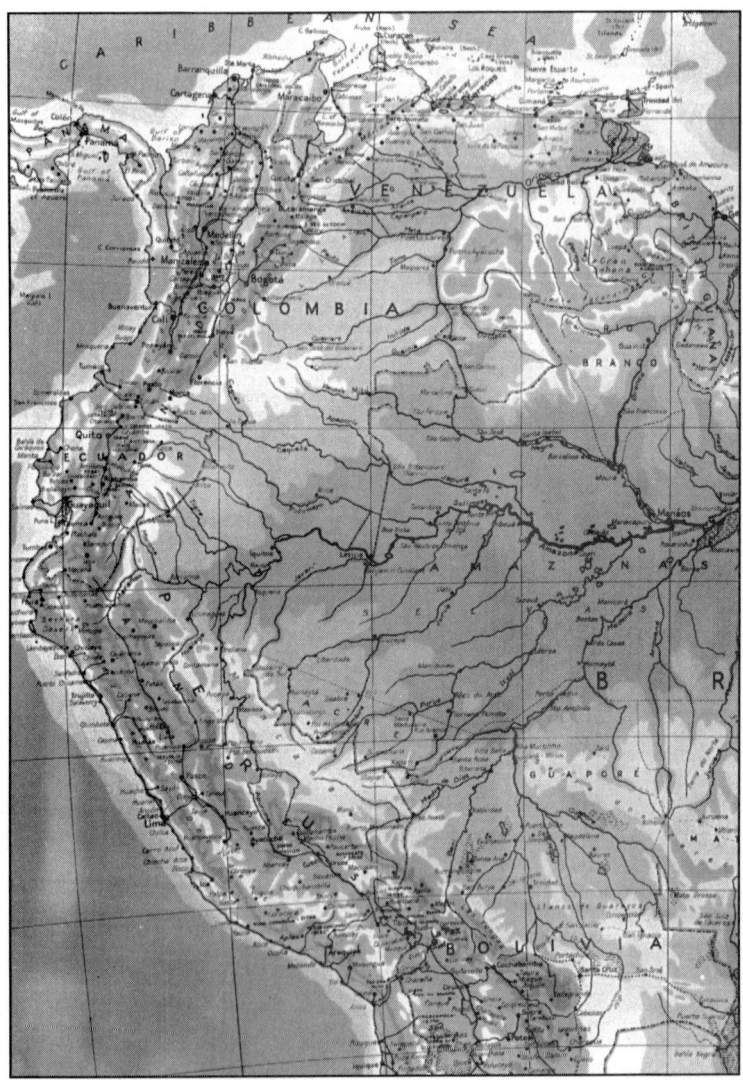

Figure 1.1: Map of northern-western South America. At the time of the Spanish conquests in S. America., New Granada was a large state incorporating present day Ecuador the western part of present day Venezuela and the northwestern part of modern Brazil.

la Condamine. The expedition was joined by a botanist Joey de Jussieu, who was already working out there and who had found and described many varieties of the cinchona trees and knew that the bark contained a bitter febrifugal material. The expedition, which lasted seven years, was bedeviled by much dispute and rivalry amongst its members and it ran into serious financial difficulties and great trouble with the Spanish authorities at Quito. In 1737 De la Condamine sent a brief description of cinchona trees to the French Academy. It was probably given to him by de Jussieu. It was from this description that Linnaeus named the genus *Cinchona*. For the next eighty years, due to a series of tragic misfortunes, this was one of only two descriptions of the cinchona trees that was available in Europe.

De Jussieu remained in South America until 1761 but all his records were stolen and destroyed by a servant. He returned to France, after working in the jungle for thirty-six years, a sick man and although he did not die until 1779 the only manuscript of his that survives, written in Latin in 1737, was first published 200 years later in 1936 by a French company which marketed quinine under the proprietary name, 'Trois Cachets'.

About the time that de Jussieu returned to Europe another botanist, José Celestino Mutis, accompanied a new viceroy to the capital of New Granada, Santa Fé de Bogotá. José Mutis, was a man of great talent. He was a physician, he was a botanist, he produced a dictionary of the native languages, wrote a treatise on mining and he sent many botanical specimens to

Linnaeus in Sweden, including specimens of *Cinchona bogotensis*. Linnaeus described Mutis as the 'prince of American botanists' and made him a member of the Academy of Sciences at Upsala. Linnaeus said that the specimens of cinchona trees that he received from Mutis were very different from those described by De la Condamine.

In 1777 a scientific mission was sent by the Spanish government to Peru and Chile. Three botanists, Ruin, Pavón and Dombey over a period of eleven years made an enormous collection of cinchona specimens. But ill luck dogged them. Their records were destroyed by fire in Peru and fifty cases containing the specimens were lost in the *San Pedro de Alcántara*. This ship was for many years thought to have been wrecked. But in 1852 the magnificent collection of cinchona barks made by the three botanists turned up in the British Museum and in retrospect it is believed the *San Pedro* must have been taken as a prize by the Royal Navy and the collection sent to the museum.

Meanwhile José Mutis did not get the support for his work which he had expected despite sending petitions to the King of Spain. But in 1782 Bishop Gongora, who had been much impressed by his scholarship, had him appointed as Chief Botanist to the Botanical Expedition of the New Kingdom of Granada and in 1791 Mutis played an important part in establishing the 'Botanical Institute of New Granada'. This Institute was the first scientific institution created in the New World. Baron Von Humboldt who visited it in 1801 was full of praise for its immense and valuable botanical collection and was impressed at the work of the thirty or so artists employed there under the Director, Francisco José de Caldas.

José Mutis was now old and although he had done so much work he had published very little. Unfortunately de Caldas was caught up in the revolutionary troubles in Granada in 1816, was condemned to death and was executed. So nothing from the Institute was published. However 104 cases of drawings, specimens and other material were sent to Spain. Most of these cases were never opened but in 1818 the botanist La Gasca was asked by the government to arrange for the publication of 122 illustration of cinchona trees in the collection. However, there was a civic revolt in Cadiz and his house was looted and all the documents were destroyed.

It was tragic that eighty years of arduous work by hard working and dedicated botanists came to so little.

The identification of the alkaloids
and attempts to cultivate cinchona

It was at this time that important advances were made by chemists. In 1816 a Portuguese naval surgeon, Dr Gómez, extracted a crude febrifuge principle from cinchona bark which he called cinchonine and four years later Pelletier and Caventou in France isolated quinine and prepared quinine sulphate. They showed that the species *Cinchona calisaya* found in Bolivia was the best source of quinine.

The Indian cascarillos or bark collectors tried to meet the increasing demand for bark but very much at the expense of the forest which was increasingly stripped of its cinchona trees. At the same time the Bolivian government in an attempt to maintain its monopoly of supply, banned the export of seeds and plants of cinchona trees, for the financial rewards which would accrue if the cinchona trees could be cultivated were already attracting European entrepreneurs.

The English botanist, Dr Weddell, a member of a French expedition to the Amazon in 1843–9 published descriptions of many species of cinchona and brought back seeds which he gave to botanists in Paris and London who, however, seemed little interested in them.

A much more determined effort to start cultivation of cinchona was made by Julius Charles Haasskarl, the superintendent of the botanic gardens in Java, in 1853. He entered Bolivia under an assumed name, stole seeds but apparently planted them inefficiently in Java so that only a few trees survived. However, when Dr Jungkuhn was appointed Director, the plantation of cinchona trees was transferred to a better site, only for it to be found that the wrong species had been chosen and that the bark contained little quinine.

In 1859 the Indian government commissioned the botanist Richard Spruce to collect seeds and plants of cinchona in Ecuador. He made a difficult journey under appalling conditions to the western slopes of Mount Chimborazo and brought back 100,000 seeds and 600 plants of the red cinchona, *Cinchona succirubra*, to Guayaquil whence they were taken to India and Ceylon by his colleague Robert Cross. The red cinchona flourished well in Ceylon and in a number of other countries including Fiji and Jamaica. Unfortunately, red cinchona contains four alkaloids, chinchonine, cinchonidine, quinidine and only a little quinine. Nevertheless, it was found worth while to produce 'Totaquine' a weakly antimalarial preparation which was produced and sold at a cost of one rupee per ounce. Mr Spruce never recovered his health after his arduous expedition, nor was he ever adequately rewarded for his efforts. Eventually after considerable hassle he received a pension of £50 a year from the India Office in London.

Charles Ledger, an English trader, with his servant Manuel Mamani had searched for but not found *Cinchona calisaya* in Bolivia in 1845. A few years later George Bachouse found the trees but was murdered by the Indians who felt that their trade in bark would be lost if Europeans stole seeds or plants. In 1865 Manuel Mamani, Ledger's servant, brought genuine *Cinchona calisaya* seeds to England and gave them to Charles Ledger. On his return to Bolivia Mamani, who was regarded by his countrymen as a traitor, was put in gaol for his efforts and was tortured and died. Ledger offered the seeds to the British government which was not quite as brisk as the Indian government and took no interest in them. Eventually he sold half of them to an Indian planter and half to a group of Dutch merchants. It was the Dutch who made the best use of these seeds. They developed plantations in Java where conditions favoured the growth of the trees. The bark of *Cinchona ledgeriana*, its new name, had a 13% content of quinine compared to the 3% content of bark from red cinchona. Thus was founded a prosperous industry in the Dutch East Indies with Amsterdam becoming the quinine market of the world.

*Commercial exploitation
and competition in the twentieth century*

By the beginning of the twentieth century the dominant world production of cinchona bark was in Java and the trade in quinine was no longer concerned with individuals: now it was committees, planters' combines, conventions and restrictive practices which dominated the scene.

Most of the bark was sent to Europe for processing but the planters in Java tried, not too successfully, to process bark in their own factory in Bandung.

The First Quinine Convention was held in 1913 and the eleven manufacturers (3 German, 4 French, 1 English, 2 Dutch and the Bandung factory) signed an agreement with the planters fixing the price of bark for five years. The outbreak of the 1914–18 war upset the arrangements, but a Second Quinine Convention was held in 1918. By 1929 there was growing anxiety about the monopoly of the Javanese production of bark for there was now increasing demand for quinine from Japan and the USA. Indeed the Americans tried to start plantations of cinchona trees in the Philippines, Haiti and Guatemala but with no great success. The response of the planters was cynical; they reduced the acreage under cultivation to increase the price and in 1934 The Cinchona Export Ordinance further restricted output to increase the price.

The rising cost of the high quality quinine from Java caused great anxiety to the Health Organisation of the League of Nations and in 1928 the League's Malaria Commission recommended that the production of Totaquine, the less efficient but much cheaper antimalarial, which was produced from the red cinchona trees which were much easier to grow and could be cultivated in many countries around the world, should be greatly increased to meet the needs of impoverished Third World countries.

It was in 1930 that an event which was to have important consequences twelve years later occurred. Systematic research at I. G. Farbenindustrie in Germany with the preparation and testing of some 12,000 compounds resulted in the production of the first effective synthetic antimalarial drug, Atabrine. When the Second World War broke out Atabrine, or mepacrine as it was called in Britain, was beginning to be used clinically, but its production was small and was mainly in Germany and the drug was not thought to be as effective as quinine.

The Romance of Remedies

The outbreak of war and its consequences

The troubles of the supply of cinchona bark in the thirties were nothing compared with the problems of the forties. In May 1940 Germany invaded Holland and all bark stored an Amsterdam was transferred to German ownership and denied to the Allies and in March 1942 the Japanese occupied Java and cut off the supply of bark completely. It was a major problem for the Allies especially for the American troops fighting in malarious areas in the Pacific and for the British troops in the Far East.

The response of the Americans was vigorous. American intelligence agencies flew red cinchona seeds from the Philippines back to the USA and cinchona plantations were planted in America and in Costa Rica while a major expedition was launched to collect bark from South America. Indeed, at least 15,000 tons of bark had been shipped back before the war had ended. At the same time the production and use of mepacrine was greatly increased and it was rapidly realised that it was as effective, if not more effective, than quinine in destroying the malarial parasites when they have invaded the red cells of the blood, an action essential for the treatment of the acute attack of malaria.

My first experience of malaria and its treatment

While I was doing my clinical training at University College Hospital, thinking that it was inevitable that I would be called up when I qualified and that it was quite likely that like my two elder brothers I would be posted abroad, I spent quite a lot of my time in the splendid Museum of Tropical Diseases that the Wellcome Trust had established in Euston Road. This stood me in good stead in rather unexpected circumstances.

One day in June 1944 I was crossing the foyer of the Medical School when the Secretary of the School came out of his office, saw me and called me over. I was to go that night to Worthing Hospital. When I got there I was welcomed by Peter Schurr, the Resident Surgical Officer, who explained to me that I was now the only resident house physician in the hospital. My predecessor had been a Portuguese doctor who, realising the invasion of Europe was about to start and that Worthing might be bombed, had understandably decided to leave. It seems amazing looking back now to realise that one year before I qualified I should have been to all extent and purposes, for I had hardly any supervision, the only doctor looking after the medical beds in that hospital – my main help being from Peter Schurr who was himself desperately busy.

A few days later a Canadian soldier was sent to the hospital with 'flu'. He was ill with a high temperature when I saw him in Casualty but within a few hours his temperature was normal. With great confidence I diagnosed malaria and sent blood to the laboratory. There was total disbelief of my diagnosis but the specimen was examined I suppose to humour me. The red

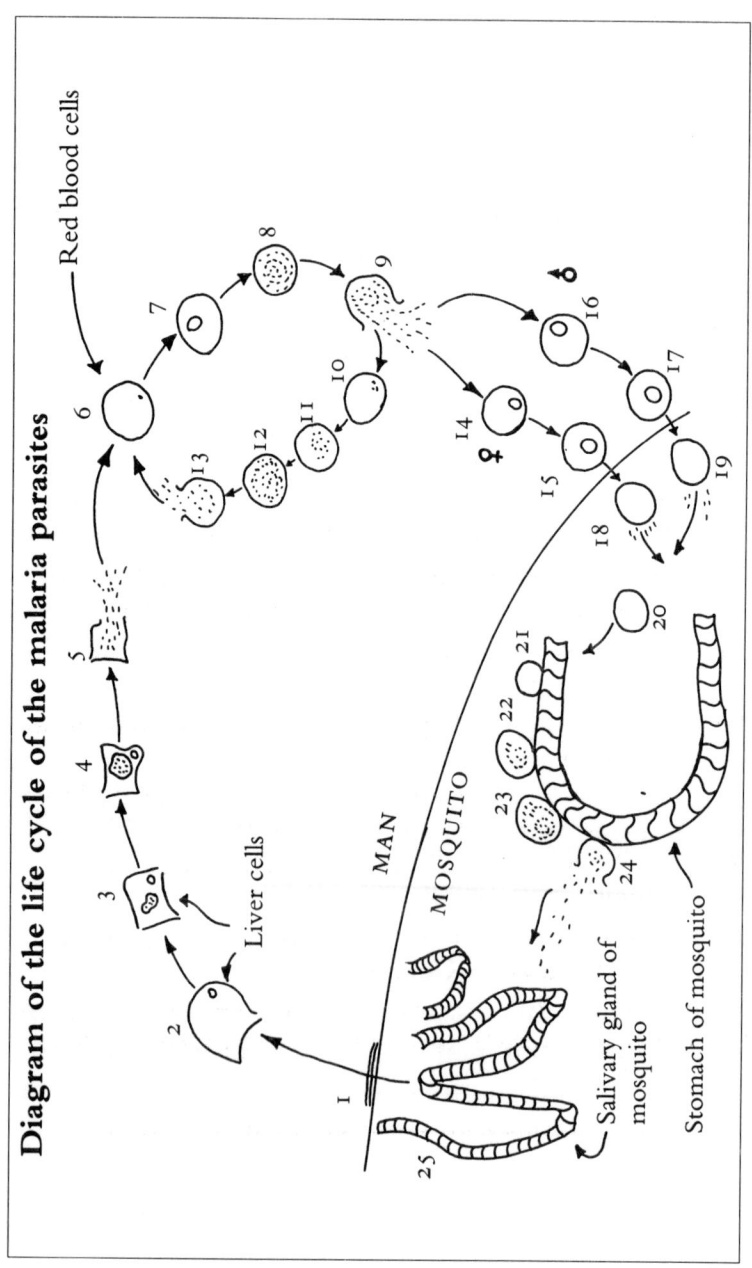

Diagram of the life cycle of the malaria parasites

Red blood cells

Liver cells

MAN

MOSQUITO

Salivary gland of mosquito

Stomach of mosquito

Quinine

Opposite: Figure 1.2.

1. When a mosquito feeds on a human, sporozoites from the salivarary gland of the mosquito are carried into human circulation.

2.–4. Sporozoites enter liver cells and mature. (exo-erythrocyte development.)

5. Merozoites released into the blood from the liver cells.

6.–8. Merozoites enter, multiply and mature in red blood cells. A few become gametocytes

9. In three or four days the red cells rupture. Patient suffers fever when merozoites are released.

10.–13. Meorzoites enter many more red cells and the cycle recurs every three or four days with resulting intermittent fever.

14.–17. Some male and female gametocytes are released and enter and mature in red cells.

18.–19. The feeding mosquito ingests red cells some of which contain gametocytes

20. Male and female gametocytes escape from red cells in the stomach of mosquito, fuse and form ookinetes.

21.–23. Ookinetes develop as oocysts in the wall of the mosquito stomach.

24. Oocysts burst and release sporozoites which migrate to the salivarary glands of the mosquito.

25. When mosquito bites another human, he is infected by sporozoites and a similar cycle starts and another human suffers from malaria.

---

cells were packed with parasites. I treated him with mepacrine.

I learnt from him that everyone in his unit, which had just returned from Tunisia, had received prophylactic mepacrine whilst in North Africa but because there was a firm belief amongst Canadian troops that mepacrine caused damage to the testes and sterility, they had stopped taking the drug as soon as they stepped onto the transport ship to return to England. Over the next two or three weeks about eighty soldiers were admitted with malaria. None was very ill but there was concern as to whether their unit would be able to proceed to France.

Chloroquine

The other important consequence of the shortage of quinine was that intensive research was instituted at the National Institute of Research at Bethedsa in the USA under the direction of Dr J. A. Shannon. This was to lead to the development of chloroquine, a very effective drug which destroys malaria parasites in red cells, and pamaquine and primaquine which are effective against the intrahepatic parasites of *Plasmodium vivax* and *P. ovale* which are responsible for recurrences of malaria after successful treatment of the acute attack.

Dr Shannon and his colleagues at the National Institute of Health at Bethedsa, Washington, USA, carried out their studies on these new antimalarial drugs in convicts in the New Jersey State Penitentiary and were subsequently criticised for this by Dr M. H. Pappworth in his book *Human Guinea Pigs*. Because I and my colleagues were also criticised, we thought entirely unfairly, by Dr Pappworth for the work we did with cardiac catheterisation in patients with rheumatic heart disease (and also incidently in ourselves), I took the opportunity when I was working in the States in 1963–4 to visit Bethesda and inquire about those studies. I think there was no doubt that this was considered a special study of strategic importance to American troops fighting in the tropics and that the volunteers regarded participation in the study as a patriotic duty. Certainly the authors of the major paper in the *Journal of Clinical Investigation* acknowledge the 'enthusiastic co-operation of the inmates of the Penitentiary', and, whatever Dr Pappworth may have thought, the prisoners were not only volunteers but were anxious to volunteer because they felt they were helping their country.

Quinine is still of value even today; given intravenously it is the drug of choice for cerebral malaria. This is caused by *P. falciparum* which causes intense parasitaemia so that 60% or 70% of red cells contain schizonts and the capillaries of the cerebral circulation are clogged with adhering parasite filled cells.

I remember many years ago late one night in Belfast admitting to my ward a pilot of British Overseas Airways. He had flown back from Cape Town to Heathrow the previous week. A defect in the aircraft wireless had caused him to make an unscheduled landing at Lagos for two or three hours. When he got back he was due for leave and came back to his home in Downpatrick. There was a lot of flu around for it was Christmas time and when he became ill it was thought he had flu, until he became unconscious. When admitted to the local hospital no one thought to ask where he had been. This is one of the really important questions that must be asked whenever someone turns up with fever of uncertain origin. He made a rapid recovery after administration of intravenous quinine.

Nowadays with the degree of parasitaemia that he had, we would almost certainly try to reduce the burden of parasitised cells by an exchange blood transfusion as well as giving quinine intravenously. And recent work has shown that the large doses of quinine given to these patients, stimulate the production of insulin and compromise the patient's recovery by causing severe hypoglycaemia; fortunately there are somatostatin analogues which can be given to attenuate the insulin releasing effects of quinine.

The present position

There were great hopes in the mid-sixties that with DDT and other organophosphate insecticides it would be possible to control the transmission of malaria by eradicating or reducing mosquito populations. It was a bitter disappointment to find that mosquitoes were able to develop resistance to these insecticides and that there were also fears that the organophosphate residues were entering human food cycles.

Even more disappointing has been the development of resistance by malaria parasites to chloroquine and other antimalarial drugs which are used in the prophylaxis and treatment of malaria, so that in many parts of the world pyrimethamine with either dapsone or sulfadoxine has to be used for prophylaxis and mefloquine or halofantrine for the treatment of falciparum malaria. It is important now for the traveller to know which prophylactic drug and which therapeutic drug is best for him to use in the country that he is to visit.

There are hopes that it may be possible to develop a vaccine against malarial parasites. This is much to be desired for malaria is still one of the 'captains of the men of death'. It is a serious health problem in more than 100 countries. It is estimated that there are some 110 million clinical cases of malaria each year and in Africa WHO estimates that between 20% and 30% of infant and childhood mortality is attributable to the disease.

The history of quinine and of our search for effective treatment of malaria is fascinating; but it is still unfinished.

CHAPTER 2

Curare

Curare and related drugs have been of special interest to me ever since I took part in experimental work on them with Professor William Mushin and had the rather daunting experience of being completely paralysed and at the same time conscious of all that was happening around me.

But first something of its fascinating history. The arrow poisons of the Indians were the subject of great interest to the first European explorers of South America and curare or urare was brought back from Guinea by Sir Walter Raleigh in 1595. There were many subsequent accounts of the way the Indians used long blow-pipes to project small arrows tipped with the poison to paralyse their prey. It was realised that the lethal action of the poison was due to its effects on the muscles of the animal but it was thought very puzzling that the meat of the poisoned animals could be eaten without any harm.

The way the Indians prepared the poison was for long shrouded in mystery for it varied from tribe to tribe, with the season, with the whim of the maker and with the ingredients available. Moreover there was much secret ritual and magic associated with it preparation. For many years only very crude preparations were available in Europe and they were classified on

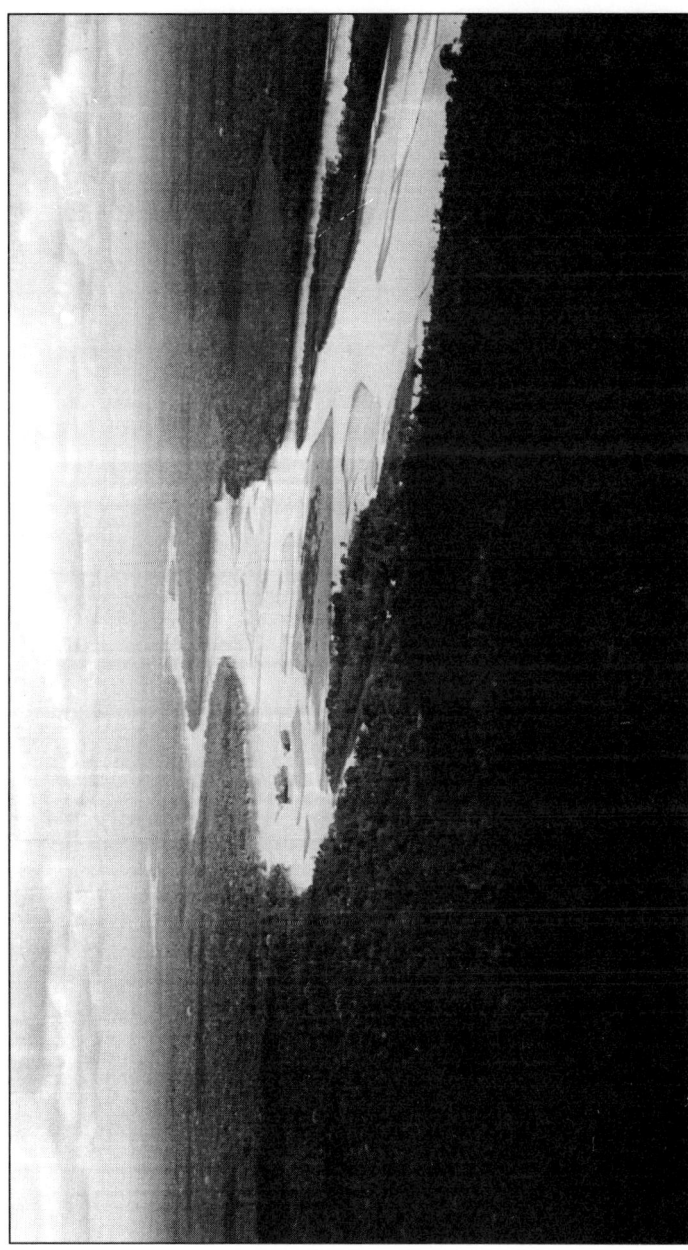

Figure 2.1: The Napo river flowing east from the Andes in Ecuador. This is an area where Indians used curare for hunting (Courtesy of Dr Philip Hugh-Jones.)

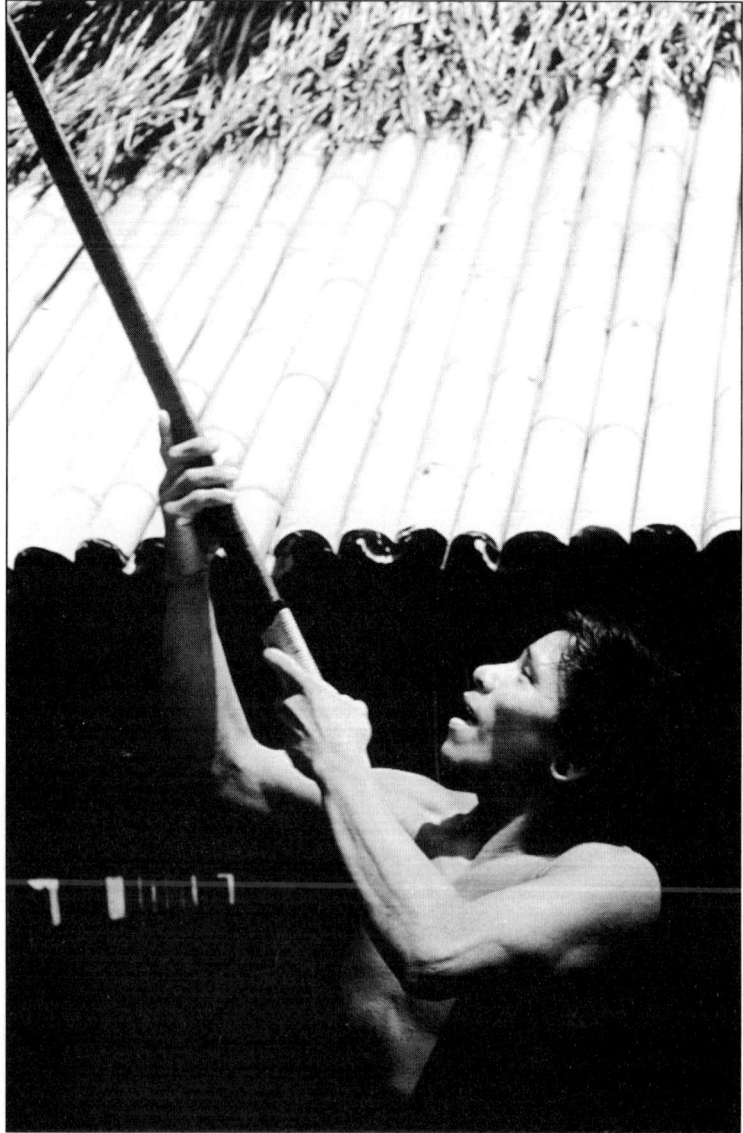

Figure 2.2: Indian hunter with blowpipe and curare-tipped arrows. He is standing in front of a hut with a bamboo roof. (Courtesy of Dr Phillip Hugh-Jones.)

the basis of the containers in which the poison was stored and transported. There were three types; tube curare (tubocurare) in bamboo tubes, calabash curare in gourds and pot curare in earthenware pots.

In 1805 Von Humboldt identified the plants which were the source of curare, or wourali as it was then known, as being either *Strychonos* or *Chondrodendron*, the latter being the source of much of the curare from Peru and Ecuador. No doubt many experimented with the crude preparations and we owe to a surgeon, Sir Benjamin Brodie, a fascinating account of the paralysis and the resuscitation of a donkey in 1814 or 1815.

A she-ass received the wourali poison in the shoulder, and died apparently in ten minutes. An incision was then made in its wind pipe, and through it the lungs were regularly inflated for two hours with a pair of bellows. Suspended animation returned. The ass held up her head, and looked around; but the inflating being discontinued, she sunk once more in apparent death. The artificial breathing was immediately recommenced, and continued without intermission for two hours. This saved the ass from final dissolution; she rose up, and walked about; she seemed neither in agitation nor pain. The wound through which the poison entered, healed without difficulty. Her constitution, however, was so severely affected that it was long in doubt if ever she would be well again. She looked lean and sickly for above a year, but began to mend the spring after, and by midsummer became fat and frisky.

The kind hearted reader will rejoice on learning that Earl Percy, pitying her misfortunes, sent her down from London to Walton Hall, near Wakefield. There she goes by the name of Wouralia. Wouralia shall be sheltered from the wintry storm and when summer comes she shall feed in the finest pasture. No burden shall be placed upon her, and she shall end her days in peace.

There is a footnote. Poor Wouralia breathed her last on the 15th of February 1839, having survived the operation nearly five and twenty years.

It was just about this time that Claude Bernard fell under the influence of the great experimental physiologist Magendie at the Collége de France in Paris. Magendie's daring though somewhat disorderly experimentation, his pitiless criticism, and his scepticism in which he included his own discoveries, made a deep impression on young Bernard. But the pupil was soon to prove a greater man than his teacher and his work and his assertion of the importance of the constancy of the internal environment (*le milieu interieur*) was to dominate physiological thinking for a century.

In 1845 Claude Bernard was given some curare from Brazil by Monsieur Pelouze. He immediately began to experiment with it. He did not however publish any of the results he obtained until 1850 when he made a brief communication to the Société de Biologie and then longer papers in 1856 and 1857.

Bernard had a very serious illness in the winter of 1862–3. The exact nature of the illness is a little uncertain. It is not unlikely that it was appendicitis for he had abdominal pain and it was suspected that he had an abdominal abscess and he suffered recurring attacks of fever. There were times in 1866–67 when his life was despaired of. but at the beginning of the illness he returned to his ancestral home at St Julien. It was here, away from his laboratory and his experiments, that he began to develop in a systematic way his views on the nature of physiological inquiry. This was to result in 1865 in one of the great books of scientific medicine, *An Introduction to the Study of Experimental Medicine*. In this book he recalls his work with curare and he describes the thinking behind his experimental work. He wrote:

We then knew nothing about the physiological action of this substance. From old observations and from the interesting accounts of Alex. von Humboldt and of Roulin and Boussingault, we knew only that the preparation of this substance was complex and difficult and that it very speedily kills an animal if introduced under the skin. But from the earlier observations, I could get no idea of the mechanism of death by curare; to get such an idea I had to make fresh observation as to the organic disturbance to which this poison might lead. I therefore made experiments to *see* things about which I had absolutely no preconceived idea. First, I put curare under the skin of a frog; it died after a few minutes; I opened it at once, and in this physiological autopsy I studied in succession what had become of the known physiological properties of its various tissues. I say physiological autopsy purposely, because no others are really instructive. The disappearance of physiological properties is what explains death, and not anatomical changes. Indeed, in the present state of science, we see physiological properties disappear in any number of cases without being able to show by our present means of observation, any corresponding anatomical change . . . Now in my frog poisoned with curare, the heart maintained its movements. The blood was apparently no more changed in physiological properties than the muscles, which kept their normal contractility. But while the nervous system had kept its normal anatomical appearance, the properties of the nerves had nevertheless completely disappeared. There were no movements either voluntary or reflex, and when the motor nerves were stimulated directly, they no longer caused any contraction in the muscles. To learn whether there was anything accidental or mistaken in this first observation, I repeated it several times and verified it in various ways; for when we wish to reason experimentally, the first thing necessary is to be a good observer and to make certain that the starting point of our reasoning is not a mistake in observation. In mammals and in birds, I found the same phenomena as in frogs and disappearance of the physiological properties of the motor system became my constant fact. Starting from this well established fact, I could then carry analysis of the phenomena further and determine the mechanism of death from curare. I still proceeded by reasoning analogous to those quoted in the above example, and, from idea to idea and experiment to experiment, I progressed to more and more definite facts. I finally reached this general proposition, that *curare causes death by destroying all the motor nerves, without affecting the sensory nerves.*

. . . In the case of curare, I instinctively reasoned in the following way: no phenomenon is without a cause, and consequently there is no poisoning without a physiological lesion peculiar or proper to the poison used; now, thought I, curare must cause death by an activity special to itself and by acting on certain definite organic parts. So by poisoning an animal with curare and by examining the properties of its various tissues immediately after death, I can perhaps find and study the lesions peculiar to it.

When I was a student we had to repeat one of Bernard's most telling experiments. If the hindleg of a frog is ligatured in a manner which deprives the limb of its circulation but allows the sciatic nerve to remain free, the injection of curare into the ventral lymph sac produces typical effects in all parts of the frog except the ligatured limb. In this unpoisoned leg, electrical stimulation of the sciatic nerve produces normal muscular contraction, whereas the muscles of the opposite poisoned limb are unresponsive to nerve stimulation.

But afferent stimulation of the poisoned leg elicits crossed reflex response in the unpoisoned limb.

It is clear that curare, to produce the observed effects, does not act centrally at the spinal cord or brain, not on the peripheral nerves but must reach the muscle to exert its effect. Further localisation of its effects is obtained by showing that the curarized muscle is still capable of responding to direct electrical stimulation and that the sciatic nerve if soaked in a solution of curare is still capable of carrying impulses. This places the site of action at the neuromuscular junction.

Over the next fifty years it was shown that curare is a competitive blocking agent acting mainly on the neuromuscular junction of skeletal muscles and to a lesser degree on autonomic ganglia. It prevents these structures responding to acetylcholine when it is released at the nerve ending in rather the same way that atropine blocks the effect of acetylcholine in smooth muscles.

Up until 1942 curare and various related alkaloids with similar properties had no valid established clinical use; attempts had been made to use the drugs in spastic paraplegia and to prevent the vicious muscular contraction which was a feature in those days of electroconvulsive therapy for severe endogenous or post parturient depression. The main reason for this failure was that the preparations of curare were so variable and unreliable. Curare was regarded by pharmacologists as one of a number of drugs which, although of no or little clinical value in the treatment of disease, were of enormous value as tools with which to explore the physiological mechanisms of the nervous system.

This was to change dramatically in 1942. Some years previously, in 1932, West had produced highly purified fractions of tubocurare which he had used, but with little success in patients with tetanus. It was Griffith and Johnson in Canada who were the first to exploit the availability of reliable standardised preparations of curare as adjuvants to anaesthetics.

When I was a student anaesthetic agents such as ether and chloroform were still being widely used, usually by the open drop technique known as 'the rag and bottle' method. I myself gave many anaesthetics by this method for my father. The real problem was that to achieve relaxation of the abdominal musculature, which was essential for all intra-abdominal surgery, the patient had to be given such a high concentration of the anaesthetic that paralysis of the medulla and respiratory arrest was a life threatening danger. The introduction of curare and the other muscle relaxants meant that the anaesthetic agent could be given in much smaller concentrations for its only purpose was to render the patient unconscious.

The other development that was to change the face of modern surgery was the arrival of the specialist anaesthetist and in our country the superb training programme for the young anaesthetists. One of the leaders in this transformation was William Mushin, the Professor of Anaesthesiology at the Welsh School of Medicine. He had trained at Oxford under Professor

Mackintosh, who had introduced tracheal intubation and closed circuit anaesthesia.

I was a young man working in the Pneumoconiosis Unit of the Medical Research Council in Cardiff and had been doing some work measuring the chest and diaphragmatic movements during respiration. The chest movements I measured with a thin rubber tube of about 1mm bore which was filled with mercury; the electrical resistance of this mercury-in-rubber transducer changed as the tube which was coiled four times around the chest, lengthened and shortened as the subject breathed. The diaphragmatic movements were measured by screening the patient radiologically and following the movements of the leaves of the diaphragm with a sliding pointer that I moved as I watched the diaphragm moving.

I was quite excited when I was approached by Mushin to ask if I would collaborate in some work which he was doing with gallamine triethiodide which was one of a number of recently synthesised curare substitutes. It appeared to have an advantage over curare in that it had a more rapid onset of action and recovery. Mushin knew that the drug paralysed the striated muscle of the limbs but was particularly anxious to determine whether the drug paralysed the muscle of the diaphragm, for the diaphragm is in some ways more like the smooth muscle of the intestines and it was known that curare did not paralyse them.

Thus it was that I found myself lying in the dark on an X-ray table with the mercury-in-rubber transducer around my chest and with Dr John Gilson screening me and recording the movements of my diaphragm. In my right hand I was holding a spring grip meter and every thirty seconds Dr Philip Hugh-Jones asked me to make as hard a grip as I could of this meter with my right hand. On my left side was Professor Mushin. He had inserted a fine catheter into a vein on the back of my left hand and he began to slowly inject gallamine. As he continued this injection my grip became weaker. Eventually however hard I tried I could not make any impression at all on the grip meter. Then I realised that I was not breathing – or at least that there were no movements of my chest, and that I was totally paralysed. I had of course been told exactly what was going to happen. I felt no fear – it was all much too interesting for that – and I could not speak. However I was completely aware of all that was happening and I could hear everything that was said. In particular I remember how comforting it was to listen to John Gilson telling me at regular intervals that despite the total paralysis of the striated voluntary muscles, 'Owen, the diaphragm is moving splendidly'. I remember just a trace of anxiety when Mushin made some comment to the effect that, 'Recovery should have started by now', because I knew that there had been reports of some muscle relaxants causing anaesthetists great anxiety as recovery might be delayed and artificial respiration, akin to that given to poor old Wourali, had to be continued for many hours.

I recovered rapidly and completely. It was an interesting experience and I would not have missed it.

CHAPTER 3

Digitalis

When I was a student digitalis was of enormous importance to all doctors who had to look after patients with heart failure. Remember that rheumatic fever, with its sequelae of valvular disease, cardiac arrhythmias and cardiac failure, was much more prevalent then than it is now. Remember, too, that we had no drugs with which to treat hypertension, a common cause of cardiac failure then as now. Remember, too, that we had no oral diuretics. We all had to know how to digitalise a patient. There were two preparation commonly prescribed, powdered digitalis leaf and tincture of digitalis. We all knew the 0. 1 gram of the powdered leaf of digitalis was the approximate equivalent of 1 ml of the tincture of digitalis.

The preparation most used in this country now is digoxin. Although it is a purified preparation and much better than the powdered leaf or the alcoholic tincture used when I was a student, it does not hold the dominant position in our *armamentarium* that its predecessors did because a number of other drugs have been developed which are effective in treating heart failure.

I am fascinated at how many lessons can be learnt about the problems of drug action, drug toxicity, bioassay, bioavailability and the general philosophy of therapy by looking back at the history of the introduction and use of digitalis.

The history of its introduction

Digitalis or foxglove is the best known of a number of plants from which drugs which have a characteristic effect on the heart can be extracted. Many of these plants are indigenous in the tropics and for centuries have been familiar to the natives of countries as diverse as the Philippines, the Malayan Archipelago, Madagascar, Lake Chad and Damaraland where they were used as arrow poisons or, more sinister because in large doses they cause severe vomiting and purging, and perhaps death, ordeal poisons – if the suspected criminal was given the drug and recovered then he or she must be a witch!

Some, such as squills and oleander, have come down to us from antiquity as medicines. They enjoyed a reputation for the treatment of diseases such as skin ulcers and 'fits'. This use can no longer be sustained and was no doubt due to the great fallacy of therapeutics, as common now as it ever was, that if someone recovers from an illness during which a medicament of some sort is given, recovery is attributed to the medicament.

Nor should it be forgotten that the line between medicine and magic is never well defined; in Europe the medieval 'doctrine of signatures' led to the use of plants which have heart shaped leaves, as foxglove has,

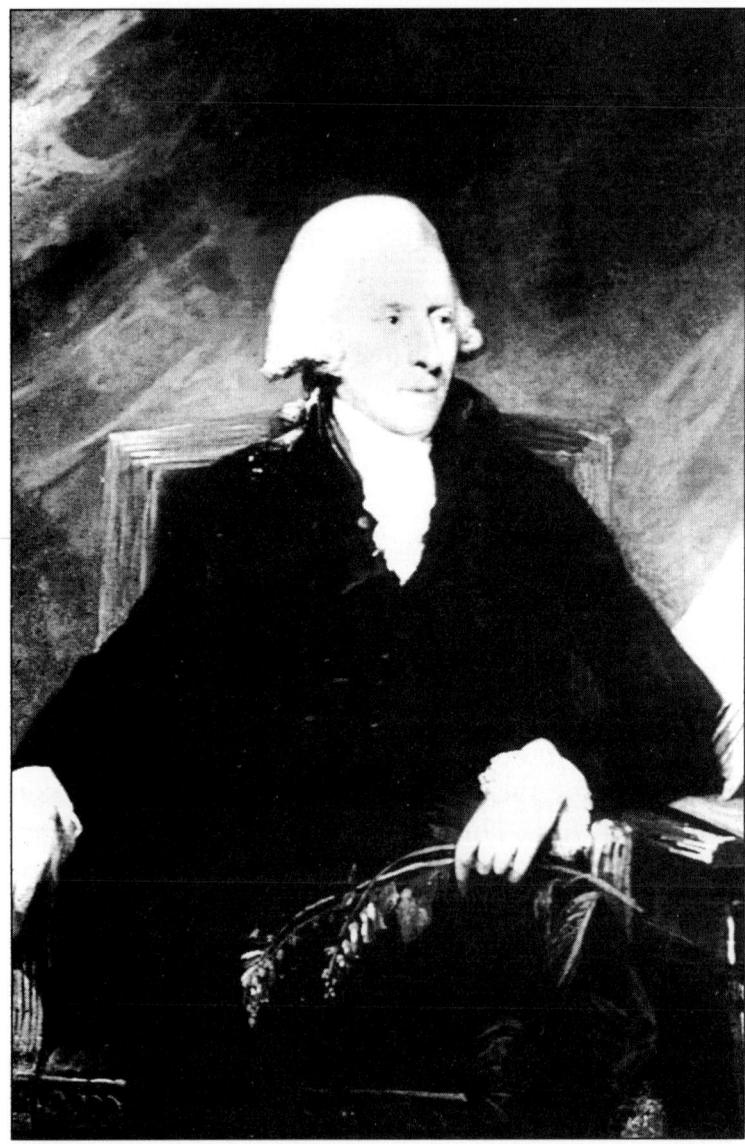

Figure 3.1: Portrait of William Withering by Von Breda. The original is in the Swedish National Museum in Stockholm. There is a copy in the Medical School of the University of Birmingham.

for heart conditions, although this may have been more for 'broken heart' than for heart disease.

The modern use of digitalis dates from 1785 when William Withering published his famous book *An Account of the Foxglove and Some of its Medical Uses.* In the book Withering tells how he came to use foxglove.

> In the year 1875 my opinion was asked concerning a family receipt for the cure of the dropsy. I was told that it had long been kept a secret by an old woman in Shropshire, who had sometimes made cures after the more regular practitioners had failed. I was informed also, that the effects produced were violent vomiting and purging; for the diuretic effects seem to have been overlooked. This medicine was composed of twenty or more different herbs; but it was not very difficult for one conversant with these subjects, to perceive that the active herb could be none other than the Foxglove.

Even today a physician who uses digitalis should read Withering's scholarly book because in it there is a clear account of many of the errors of digitalis administration which are still seen today. For six years when I was Dean of the Faculty of Medicine and Dentistry at the University of Birmingham, I sat at my desk in the Dean's room with Withering looking down on me from his portrait with a foxglove in his hand and a rather anxious expression on his face in case I made any errors!

Diagram of the chambers of the heart
(Arrows indicate direction of blood flow.)

Superior vena carva – Blood returns from all parts of the body to the right artium via the superior and inferior venae cavae.

Pulmonary Trunk – Blood is ejected through the pulmonary arteries to the lungs, is oxygenated and returns to the left venticle.

Ascending aorta

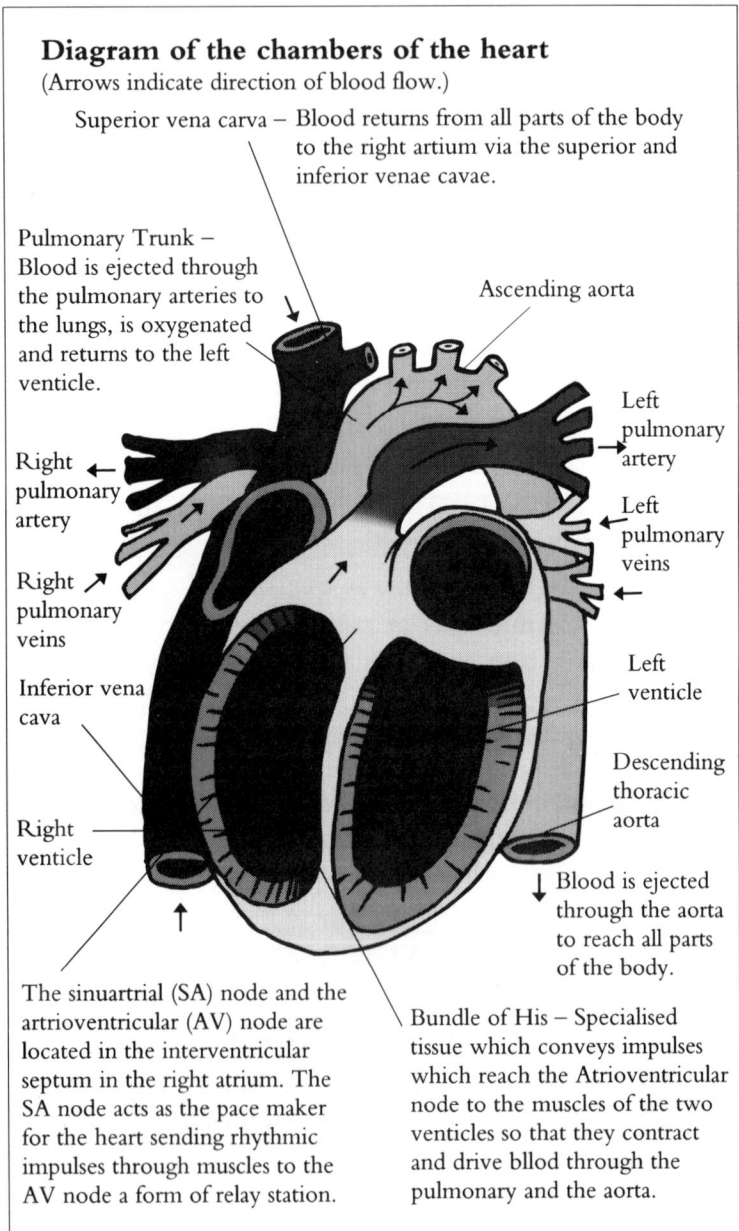

Right pulmonary artery

Left pulmonary artery

Left pulmonary veins

Right pulmonary veins

Inferior vena cava

Left venticle

Descending thoracic aorta

Right venticle

Blood is ejected through the aorta to reach all parts of the body.

The sinuartrial (SA) node and the artrioventricular (AV) node are located in the interventricular septum in the right atrium. The SA node acts as the pace maker for the heart sending rhythmic impulses through muscles to the AV node a form of relay station.

Bundle of His – Specialised tissue which conveys impulses which reach the Atrioventricular node to the muscles of the two venticles so that they contract and drive bllod through the pulmonary and the aorta.

Digitalis

The site of action of digitalis

Although Withering recognised that the drug had 'a power over the motion of the heart to a degree yet unobserved in any other medicine', he did not associate this effect with its value in the treatment of dropsy and for many years foxglove was regarded as a diuretic drug and believed to act on the kidney. However in patients in cardiac failure without oedema or serous effusions, the drug did not cause diuresis. Nor did it do so in patients with dropsy due to causes other than cardiac failure.

It is thought that Withering's contemporary, John Ferriar, was the first physician to recognise that it was its effect on the heart which was its most important action, and by the end of the last century it was widely realised that the increased urinary output that may follow the administration of digitalis was a consequence of increased cardiac output and increased blood flow to the kidney.

Opposite: Figure 3.2

Diagram of the heart and the circulation of the blood. If the muscle of the auricles is damaged by rheumatic fever or coronary artery disease, the normal wave of contraction is replaced by irregular contraction of the muscle fibres of the auricles or 'fibrillation'. Instead of 60 impulses a minute reaching the AV node, as many as 600 impulses may reach it. It responds irregularly about 160–180 times per minute and thus ventricular contractions are frequent, irregular and inefficient in driving blood around the circulation causing heart failure.

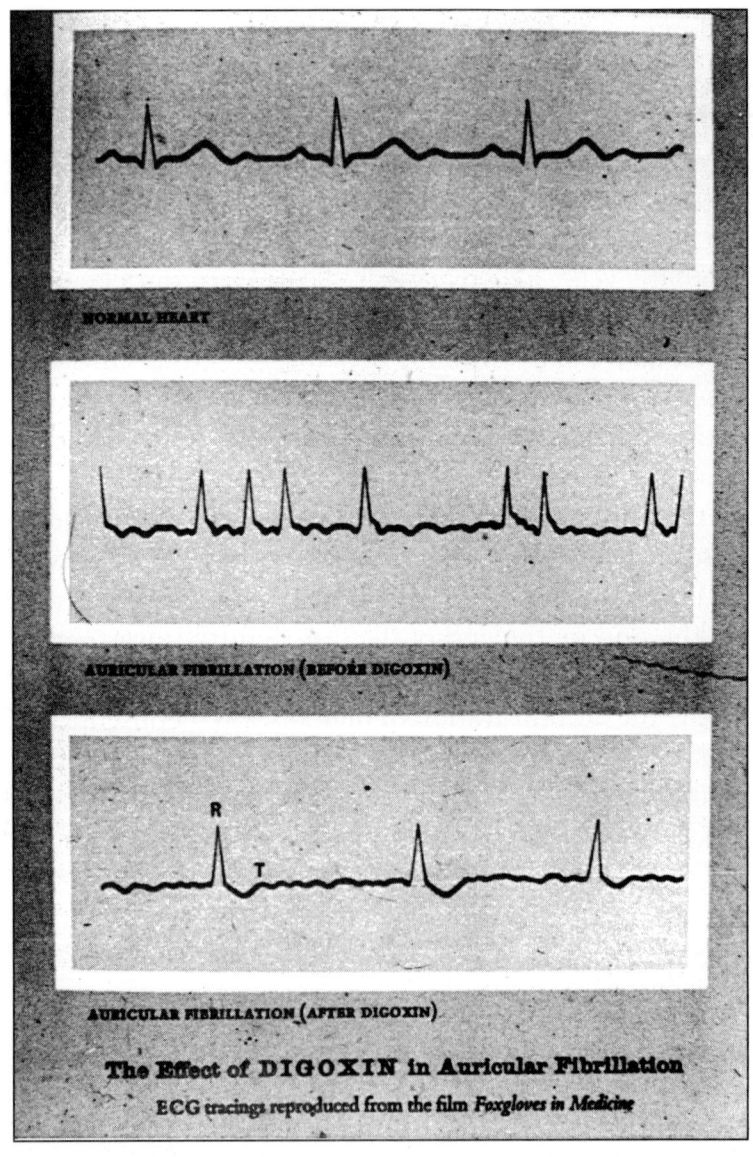

NORMAL HEART

AURICULAR FIBRILLATION (BEFORE DIGOXIN)

AURICULAR FIBRILLATION (AFTER DIGOXIN)

The Effect of DIGOXIN in Auricular Fibrillation
ECG tracings reproduced from the film *Foxgloves in Medicine*

Digitalis

Digitalis and auricular fibrillation

Auricular fibrillation was first recognised in man in 1901 by Cushny and Edmunds. They reported their description of the condition and the way in which it led to rapid and irregular ventricular contractions in 1906 but it was received with much doubt by their contemporaries until it was confirmed by the new electrocardiographic methods in the hands of Rothberger and Winterberg (1909) and Lewis (1910).

When I was a student at University College Hospital, London, during the war, I was a medical clerk on Sir Thomas Lewis's firm and I remember that one afternoon I and another student were attending his clinic in the Out-Patient Department, which was in a basement room on the Gower Street side of the building. While he was examining a patient a steam roller passed down the street above us making a frightful noise so that it was impossible for Lewis to listen to the patient's heart with his stethoscope. While he waited for the noise to cease he told us that it was in an adjacent room that he had first set up the primitive Einthoven string galvanometer and made his first electrocardiographic recordings of a patient with auricular

---

Opposite: Figure 3.3
Electrocardiographic records of cardiac contractions. In the normal heart the contractions are regular. If there is auricular fibrillation the ventricle of the heart beats rapidly and irregularly. If digitalis is given the ventricle still beats irregularly, but much slower and therefore much more efficiently as a pump circulating the blood.

fibrillation. In those days of horse traffic, Gower street was very busy during the day and he had had to come in late at night in order to make records which were not upset by the vibrations caused by the iron-bound cart wheels passing down the street.

In auricular fibrillation the auricles of the heart cease to contract normally; instead their walls are in a fine tremor due to uncoordinated muscle fibre contractions. They lose their ability to propel blood into the ventricles and the flow of blood through them to the ventricles is maintained by the pressure in the great veins. Five or six hundred electrical impulses a minute are generated within the walls of the quivering auricles and fall like a shower each minute on the auriculoventricular node and the bundle of His. These structures are unable to transmit all the impulses to the ventricles but allow a certain number to pass at irregular intervals. The ventricles therefore respond with fast, irregular and inefficient contractions usually beating about 120–180 times a minute.

It was James Mackenzie, a physician working in Burnley, who in 1911 showed that digitalis, by interfering with the conduction of impulses from the AV node to the ventricular muscle along the Purkinje tissue of the bundle of His, slowed the ventricular response and by giving the ventricles time to fill with blood between their beats improved the output of the heart.

Over the years there has continued to be controversy between those like Cushny, Lewis and Mackenzie, who believed that the dominant virtue of digoxin was that it improved the cardiac output by this effect in patients with auricular fibrillation and those who believed that digitalis and the other cardiac glycosides had an important effect direct on cardiac muscle fibres enhancing their power of contraction and thus increasing cardiac output even if there was normal cardiac rhythm present.

This latter view was held by Wenkebach (1910), Harrison *et al* (1931), and Gold and Cattell (1940). When I was working on a fellowship in New York in the early 1950s I had the opportunity of working with Dr Cournand and his two lady colleagues, Drs Harvey and Ferrer at Bellevue Hospital. In 1949 'Les girls', as Cournand always called them, had made measurements of the cardiac output at rest in patients with normal cardiac rhythm using the newly introduced technique of cardiac catheterization. They had found a small and not very convincing rise in cardiac output in patients given digitalis in whom the cardiac output at rest was decreased. But there was no evidence of any improvement if the cardiac output was normal. It was some years later before it was shown that digitalis did increase the cardiac output if it was given to patients with auricular fibrillation.

Biological assay

One of the problems of using the older preparations of digitalis was that the content of cardiac glycosides in foxgloves varied from season to season due to the changes in rainfall, temperature or soil. This led to the development by Houghton in the USA in 1898 of a method of measurement that was based on measuring the effects of the drug on animals which he called a 'pharmacological assay' and which is now known as a 'biological assay'. The principle of a biological assay is that the potency of a new preparation is compared with that of an existing standard preparation. Houghton's assay was based on the amount of the new preparation that had to be given to kill frogs compared with the amount of the standard preparation that was needed to do this. Houghton's method was soon adopted by pharmaceutical manufacturers in the USA and then by Swiss, English and German firms. In the USA the assay was later based on a similar comparison made in the cat but this was eventually replaced by a similar method in anaesthetized pigeons.

An international standard for digitalis was eventually established under the aegis of the League of Nations. The International Digitalis Unit was defined as the potency of 0. 1 gram of the International Digitalis Standard Powder kept in the Institute of Medical Research of the Medical Research Council at Hampstead in London. Although digoxin was crystallised and its molecular structure characterised in 1930 by Dr Sydney Smith of the Wellcome Foundation, biological assay of digitalis was still of importance to the drug industry until after the 1939–45 war.

Biological assay was and still is of very great importance for the standardisation of vaccines for which stoichiometric analysis (measurement of atomic weights) is impossible. The mathematical methods used in biological assay owe much to Dr Gaddum who worked with Dr Trevan at the Wellcome Physiological Research Laboratories in Beckenham. The sigmoid curve that relates the dose to the biological effect is converted to a straight line either by using logarithmic probability paper or by plotting the logarithm of the dose against mortality on a probit scale.

The administration of digitalis and its problems

There have always been problems in the administration of digitalis to patients. They were familiar to Withering and they exist today. They stem from the fact that until a 'therapeutic concentration' of a cardiac glycoside had been achieved the drug had little effect on cardiac function; unfortunately this therapeutic concentration is only a little lower than the concentration of the drug at which the symptoms and signs of toxicity begin to occur, nausea, vomiting, coupling of beats, arrhythmias and ultimately heart block.

The problem for the physician is how to reach the therapeutic concentration and yet avoid serious toxicity. I found this fairly easy in patients in heart failure with auricular fibrillation. I usually used oral digoxin. I gave doses of o. 75 mg every twelve hours until the ventricular heart rate had decreased to 90 or 100 per minute. Then I reduced the dose to a 'maintenance dose' of o. 25 mg once or twice a day. The slower rate of beating, the longer period of cardiac filling and the consequent improved cardiac output might be accompanied by a diuresis, but often, if I gave a thiazide diuretic at the same time as the digoxin because there was oedema present, I would prescribe potassium salts, for the loss of potassium in the urine might otherwise increase the likelihood of digoxin causing arrhythmias. Over the next few days I would adjust the maintenance dose so that the ventricular rate would be 75–80 per minute.

In patients who were not in auricular fibrillation it was, in my experience, much more difficult to digitalise a patient; it was usually a matter of continuing the digitalisation dose until there were signs of toxicity such as nausea and vomiting and then reducing the dose to a rather arbitrary maintenance dosage.

When I first went to Belfast I was rather comforted to find that even experienced cardiologists had the same difficulty as I did and my colleague Dr Evan Fletcher developed a test using acetylstrophanthidin, a very short acting cardiac glycoside, with which it could be shown whether a patient was receiving too much or too little digoxin. It was not an easy test to carry out and was never widely used.

It is a measure of the difficulty that doctors have in digitalising a patient correctly that when Dr Hurwitz and I carried out one of the earliest studies ever done on the prevalence of adverse reactions to drugs in the Belfast City Hospital in 1963, we found digitalis was the most frequent cause of drug induced adverse reactions.

Digitalis

Plasma digoxin levels

Towards the end of 1968 it became possible for the first time to measure plasma digoxin concentrations with a sensitive radio-immuno assay. There were initially great hopes that this would help clinicians to adjust the dose of digoxin for patients so that a therapeutic concentration could be accurately achieved and toxicity avoided. It has been a sad disappointment to find that the clinical effects of digoxin in individual patients do not relate closely to the plasma levels, perhaps because factors such as the intracellular potassium concentration alter the cardiac response to digoxin. However it has been of some value to find that the toxic effects of digoxin are most unlikely to occur if the digoxin plasma levels are below 2 nanograms/ml.

By a strange quirk of coincidence it was research workers investigating the possibility of using measurements of plasma digoxin concentrations as a guide to dosage who first detected what became known as the 'bioavailability crisis'. It was May 1972. They were measuring the plasma levels of digoxin in patients who were receiving a regular dose of Lanoxin, the Burroughs Wellcome brand of digoxin. To their horror and quite unexpectedly they found that batches of the Lanoxin tablets made after May 1972 produced in patients twice the plasma levels of the tablets manufactured before May 1972, although all the tablets had the same content of digoxin.

The Romance of Remedies

Bioavailability of digoxin: the 1972 crisis

The bioavailability of a drug is the rate and extent to which it is absorbed from a given pharmaceutical preparation and becomes available at its site of action. It has been shown that the bioavailability of many drugs may be influenced by the way they are formulated and prepared. It may change if the fillers, buffers, solvents, or stabilisers are altered by the manufacturer and sometimes it will change if the tablet compression or the size of the granules in the tablet is changed when tablets are made. These changes in bioavailability are seldom of very great clinical consequence but they are important with some drugs like digoxin or warfarin for which very precise dosage is important.

I was a member of the Committee on Safety of Medicines at the time that the report of the changes in bioavailability of digoxin were reported. The position looked hazardous. A calculation suggested that a third of all patients receiving o. 5 mg/day of digoxin might be in jeopardy of suffering digitalis toxicity if they continued to take Lanoxin tablets because their plasma levels of digoxin would exceed 2 nanograms/ml.

Warnings about this potentially dangerous change in the Lanoxin tablets was immediately sent out to all doctors in Great Britain. but much to our surprise the issue of Lanoxin tablets with such greatly increased bioavailability did not seem to have caused very much trouble. There was no great increase in the number of patients suffering seriously from digitalis toxicity. I suspect that this may have been due to the fact that doctors would have adjusted the dose of digoxin downwards as soon as the early signs of digitalis toxicity, nausea and vomiting, occurred. Indeed the most serious problem, as so often in modern medicine, was that a number of patients with heart disease were frightened by the misleading and sensational reports in the media and stopped taking their tablets with consequent return of their heart failure.

The use of cardiac glycosides in Europe

In 1963 I started to look at the prescribing of medicines by doctors in Northern Ireland, work which was made possible because the data of all prescriptions was recorded so that pharmacists could be paid. In 1969 at a meeting held by WHO in Oslo, this work was extended to Norway and Sweden. It was later extended to other countries but it was not possible to extend it to England until the mid-1980s.

In order to carry out such studies it was necessary to have a unit of drug use because different cardiac glycosides are used in the different countries in Europe and the different glycosides such as digoxin, digitoxin and oubain are given in very different doses. For this purpose we devised the DDD or Defined Daily Dose per 1000 people in the community, per day.

It was found that the use of cardiac glycosides varied greatly in different countries and much the greatest use was in Germany. Studies led by my colleague Professor Hans Friebel of Heidelberg showed that this large use

CARDIAC GLYCOSIDES 1977-1979

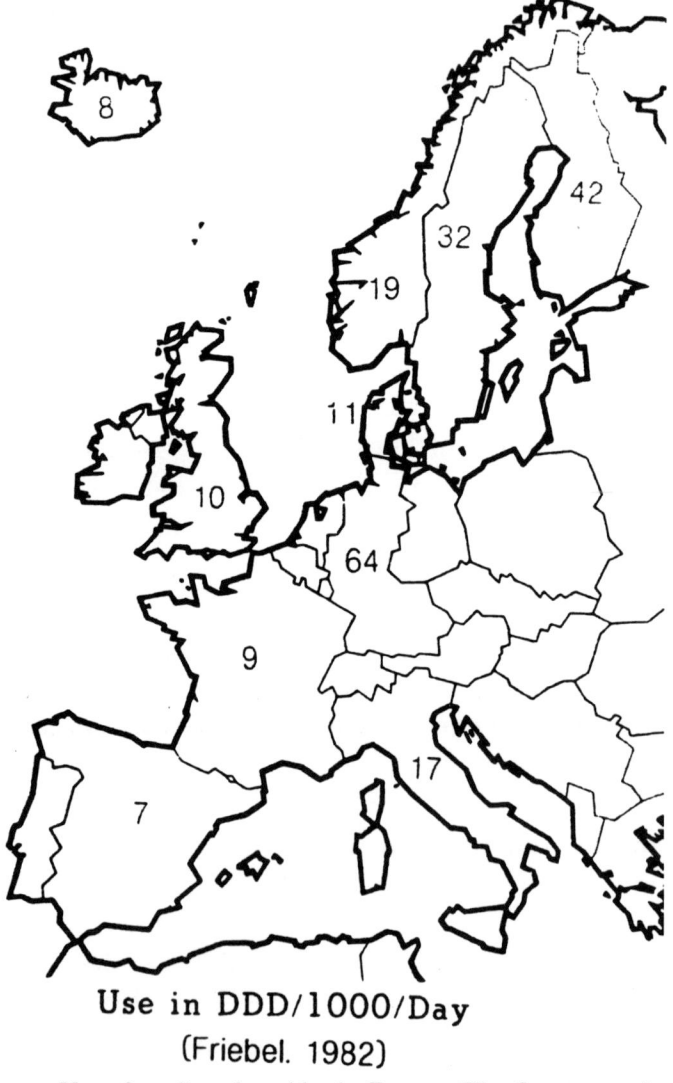

Use in DDD/1000/Day
(Friebel. 1982)

Figure 3.4: Use of cardiac glycocides in Europe. The figures are the number of doses prescribed, per 1000 people in the population, per month

of cardiac glycosides in Germany is due to a belief held by German doctors that the 'aged' heart of anyone over the age of 60 benefits from the use of a 'heart tonic', and therefore small dose of cardiac glycosides, usually digitoxin or oubain or strophanthin, are widely prescribed. In Britain, the USA and Canada it is considered inappropriate to prescribe a cardiac glycoside unless there is a good therapeutic reason such as auricular fibrillation or cardiac failure.

That prescribing of medicines in different countries differs because doctors have different ideas about the therapeutic effectiveness of a drug or about what constitutes disease does not surprise me. Some time ago Roger Bannister drew attention to the fact that there is a high prevalence in most European countries of 'low blood pressure'. This is a 'disease' often diagnosed by practitioners on the Continent, which appears to be absent in the UK. But I suspect the 'disease' exists just as much here as on the Continent but here it is diagnosed as 'nerves' and is treated as inappropriately with tranquillisers as I suspect 'low blood pressure' is treated with drugs in Germany.

Conclusion

As I look back on the history of the introduction and use of digitalis I cannot help reading with more insight than previously the words of William Withering:

The foxgloves leaves with caution given
Another proof of favouring heaven
Will happily display.
The rapid pulse it can abate,
The hectic flush can moderate
And, blest by Him whose will is fate
May give a lengthen'd day.

CHAPTER 4

Sulphonamides

People forget and it is difficult now for me to explain just how exciting it was when the first sulphonamides arrived. For the patient, or for anxious parents or relatives, some of the terrors of scarlet fever, meningitis and pneumonia were allayed. For the doctor it was wonderful to have available effective remedies where previously there had been none. For the pharmacologist it meant a total reappraisal of his discipline; no longer were drugs predominantly valuable tools with which to explore the physiological mechanisms of the body or of useful but limited use in alleviating suffering. Suddenly they were effective curative agents. The physician could cure as effectively as the surgeon. For the public and the media they were the new twentieth-century magic.

The sulphonamides have a special place in my life. They saved my father's life when I was a boy and it was the explosion in pharmaceutical development that their arrival heralded that created the need for a new sort of pharmacologist and gave me a career when I grew up.

The Romance of Remedies

Discovery

For a while the tired waves vainly breaking
Seem here no painful inch to gain
Far back through creeks and inlets making
Comes silent flooding in the main. A. H. CLOUGH 1819–61

In the early 1890s Paul Ehrlich, pathologist and founder of modern immunology, was working in the State Institute for the Investigation and Testing of Sera at Berlin. He was a contemporary of the histologists Weigert and Heidenhahn. They had shown how the stains that they used in their work were picked up differentially by different tissues and cells and this specificity of stains was no doubt in Ehrlich's mind when he conceived the idea that it might be possible to produce drugs which when given to the patient would damage the parasites or bacteria that were causing an illness but not hurt the patient; a concept given the imaginative description of 'magic bullets'.

Quinine seemed to be just such a chemotherapeutic remedy for malaria and Ehrlich sought to develop other potent remedies. He tried methylene blue, but although it stained malaria parasites dark blue it did not seem to be at all effective therapeutically. More successful were his studies with the Japanese bacteriologist, Shiga, with trypan red which had a definite curative action on laboratory induced infections of rodents with trypanosomes, the cause of the debilitating 'sleeping sickness' in central Africa.

A more effective antitrypanosomal drug, atoxyl, was

developed in Liverpool by Thomas and Breinl. Atoxyl was an arsenical compound and as perhaps its name suggests, turned out to be too toxic to use in humans. But it led Ehrlich and his colleagues to develop other organic arsenical drugs like arsphenamine and neo-arsphenamine which were partially effective in the treatment of syphilis.

Despite great endeavour no other drugs effective against bacterial disease were developed and in the 1920s and early 1930 it was widely accepted that the future of the treatment of bacterial infections in man lay in the development of vaccines and antisera.

The first azo-dyestuffs containing sulphonamide and substituted sulphonamide groups were prepared in 1908 by the Viennese chemist P. Gelmo and over the next few years the great German Chemical firm, IG Farbenindustrie, synthesised a number of other azo-dyes containing sulphonamides. These dyes had the great advantage of being colour-fast because they combined with the proteins of wool or silk.

It is said that the idea that these dyes might be of use as medicaments was first conceived by Professor Hörlein. He was later to be tried but acquitted at Nuremberg on the charge of supplying the SS with Zyklon-B gas which was used in the death chambers of the concentration camps. Several of the dyes, pyridium, scarlet red, chrysoidine and serenium, were shown to have slight bactericidal effects *in vitro* and were used as wound dressings or urinary antiseptics. None was very effective.

Gerhard Domagk was Research Director for Bayer in the company's Chemotherapeutic Research Laboratory at Elberfeld in the late 1920s. Brought up in the tradition of Ehrlich, Behring, the discoverer of the cause of diphtheria, and Koch, who identified the tubercle bacillus, he saw promise in two approaches to the control of bacterial infections; either to enhance the natural defence powers of the body by vaccines or sera or to damage the invading bacteria.

He and his colleagues Mietzch and Klarer were much influenced by the work that they had done in developing the antimalarial drug Atebrin (mepacrine in this country), for which they had used finches with induced avian malarian infections. They developed a technique of infecting mice with virulent streptococci which normally caused their death within forty-eight hours. It was Domagk's brilliant inspiration to test Prontosil, which was completely ineffective against bacteria in the test tube, in his mice which resulted in the surprising discovery of its therapeutic value in 1932.

Very wisely further work was done to confirm this finding before their work was published in the *Deutsche Medizinische Wochenschrift* on Friday 15 February 1935, with two other papers reporting the successful treatment of streptococcal infections in man. Many years later I learnt that one of the first patients ever treated with Prontosil was Domagk's 4-year-old daughter who had a septic wound and life threatening septicaemia.

These three short papers began a new era in the treatment of bacterial infection and four years later

Sulphonamides

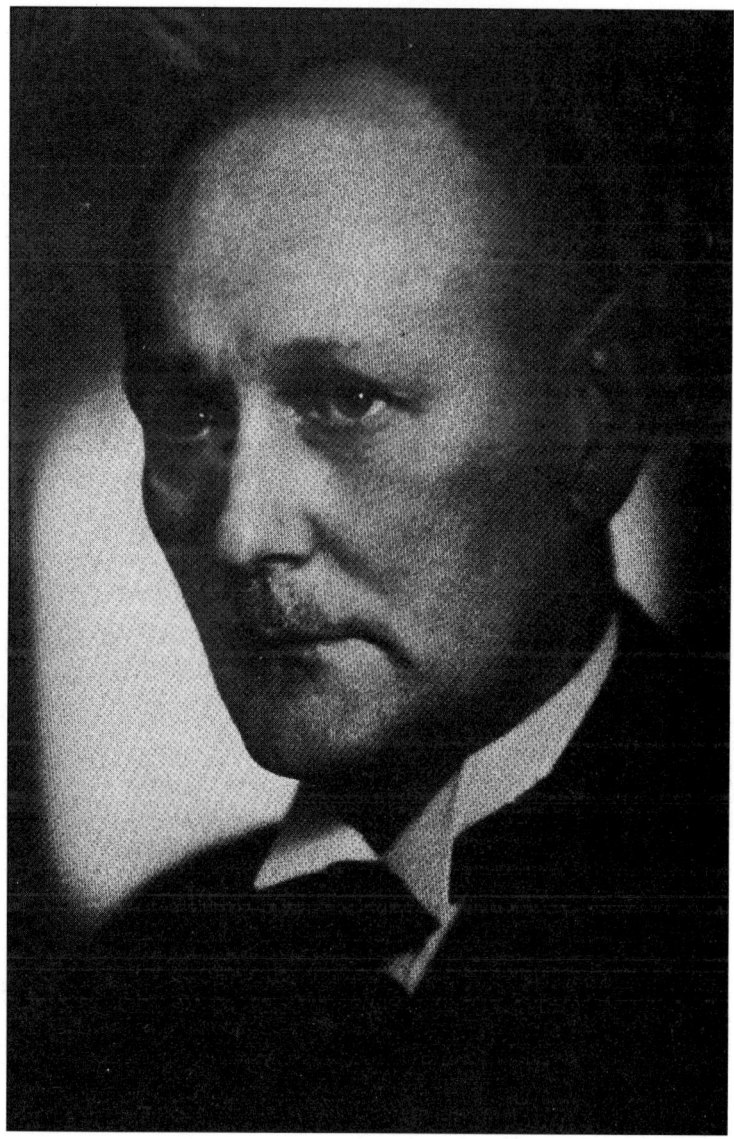

Figure 4.1: Dr Domagk, awarded Nobel prize for his work on Prontosil

Domagk was awarded a Nobel prize 'for the discovery of the antibacterial activity of Prontosil'. Poor Domagk; Hitler had ruled that no German was allowed to accept a Nobel Prize because the Nobel Prize for Peace had been awarded to Carl von Ossietsky who had expressed strong adverse criticism of the Nazi regime. When the award was made in 1939 the German radio and press were not allowed to announce the news and a few days after Domagk had written to the Nobel Committee to thank them for the recognition of his research and to express his desire to go to Stockholm to receive the prize, he was questioned by the Gestapo and arrested. He was discharged from prison a week later but prohibited from travelling outside Germany. Not until 1947, eight years later, was Domagk able to receive the diploma and the gold medal from the hands of the King of Sweden, although rather perversely his prize money had been forfeited in accordance with the by-laws of the Nobel Committee.

Further developments

Almost as soon as the effectiveness of Prontosil rubra had been proclaimed, four workers in the Pasteur Institute in Paris, M and Mme Trefouël, Nitti and Bovet showed that in the tissues of the host the dye was split at its azo linkage (N=N) and that its chemotherapeutic properties were due to the resultant sulphanilamide molecule. I cannot help feeling that the Bayer chemists should have foreseen that this was likely; it certainly was to cost their firm dearly for the patent rights for Prontosil were immediately devalued.

In England Dr G. A. H. Buttle working in the Wellcome Laboratories in Beckenham confirmed the effectiveness of Prontosil in streptococcal infections of mice. Quite independently, stimulated by a postcard sent from Paris in August 1935 by his friend Claude Lillingston, Leonard Colebrook who was a bacteriologist at that time working in the Inoculation Department at St Mary's Hospital, London, obtained Prontosil with some difficulty from Bayer. His experiments on mice were getting nowhere but Buttle came to his rescue and supplied him with strains of streptococci which were more virulent than those he had been using.

Having satisfied himself of its efficacy in streptococcal infections in mice, Colebrook used the drug to treat patients with puerperal fever at Queen Charlotte's Hospital for Mothers and Children. The results were dramatic and the two papers by Colebrook and Kenny in the *Lancet* in 1936 aroused the interest of the world.

Leonard Colebrook was later appointed as Director of the MRC Burns Unit first in Glasgow and then at the Accident Hospital in Birmingham. He had retired by the time I went to Birmingham but I heard him lecture. A slim athletic-looking man who had made a major contribution to the reduction of serious burn accidents by leading a campaign to reduce the flammability of children's clothes.

Dr Buttle served in the RAMC in the war and was posted in 1943 as a consultant to the military hospital at Alexandria. Quite characteristically and in total disregard of army regulations, he arranged for one of his colleagues in America to supply a substantial quantity of a newly synthesised sulphonamide, sulphaguanidine, at that time being made from seabird guano collected from Caribbean rocks. The 8th Army had this highly effective non-toxic antidysenteric drug before El Alamein. It may have played a part in giving them the edge over their opponents. His CO ignored a War Office instruction to reprimand Buttle for not acting through official channels! After the war Buttle became Professor of Pharmacology at the School of Pharmacy of London University in Bloomsbury Square. I met him many years later. By that time he had become deaf and all conversation with him had to be conducted as if at sea in heavy weather. His foghorn voice was a feature of all meeting of the British Pharmacological Society until he died in 1983.

In November 1936 my father who was a surgeon, pricked his finger while operating on a patient with a septic peritonitis. A fulminating infection of his hand was accompanied by an ascending vicious lymphangitis of his forearm and arm, a high fever and a septicaemia. I can remember that we children had to creep around the house and keep unaccustomedly quiet and amongst the grown-ups there was an oppressive gloom. Prontosil rubra was obtained, I think from St Mary's Hospital, and given to my father. I know no details – I was too young – but I can remember vividly the extraordinary astonishment and elation of the grown-ups when father started to get better within the next forty-eight hours; it became clear to us children that they had thought he was going to die.

The magic powder

The next time I met up with sulphanilamide was in September 1939 just after war had been declared. The big mental hospital at Whitchurch on the outskirts of Cardiff had been converted into a military hospital, as indeed it had been in the First World War for it had the great advantage that ambulance trains could be shunted into a siding adjacent to the hospital which made the transfer of stretcher cases easy.

My father had received an urgent call to the hospital to see a corporal who had a perforated gastric ulcer. This unfortunate man had been called up as a reservist to a camp near Brecon. On arrival he and his colleagues were given a splendid army meal of steak, chips and peas followed by spotted dick (suet pudding with currents). Shortly afterwards the corporal felt very poorly with severe epigastric pain. He went to his tent and lay in agony all night. In the morning the Regimental Sergeant Major showed little sympathy and he had to get up and was marched off to the sick parade. Whilst waiting to be seen he collapsed, was attended immediately by one of the medical officers and was sent to Whitchurch by ambulance.

When father saw him he had all the signs of a severe peritonitis and at operation, at which I assisted, we picked out pieces of steak, peas and chips from the peritoneal cavity and then sutured an enormous gastric perforation. My father was worried that after such massive soiling of the peritoneal cavity there would be fulminating and probably fatal sepsis. He thought this might be held at bay by the topical application of sulphanilamide powder into the peritoneal cavity.

The theatre orderly was a RAMC sergeant and he opened a sterile packet of sulphanilamide powder and attempted to pour the powder into the abdomen through the incision, which my father intended to suture with a large drain at its lower end. However the powder did not run very freely and to our horror the sergeant leant forward and blew the remainder of the powder into the abdomen. When my father tried to stop him the sergeant looked up in amazement and said, 'But its sulphanilamide, sir! It kills all the bugs.' To him, and indeed to most of the public and many journalists, sulphanilamide was magic; the sergeant found it very difficult to accept that he had done anything that was at all wrong.

The sulphonamide era

Numerous derivatives of sulphanilamide were synthesised and when I started my clinical training at University College Hospital, London, in 1942 their use dominated the clinical treatment of infectious diseases. One of the most widely used was sulphapyridine which was made by May and Baker. It was shown by Lionel

Whitby to be extremely effective against pneumococci and was marketed as M&B 693, the firm's code number for the drug. Overnight this put an end to extremely interesting and quite promising work on anti-pneumococcal sera in the treatment of pneumonia.

Sulphapyridine was to achieve a peculiar fame. In December 1943 when Churchill, on his way back from meeting Stalin, fell ill with pneumonia in Tunisia, he was treated with sulphapyridine by his physician, Lord Moran. Churchill's account of his treatment was couched in suitable military terms; 'This admirable M & B from which I did not suffer any inconvenience, was used at this earliest moment and after a week's fever the intruders were repulsed.'

I met Lionel Whitby in rather embarrassing circumstances in 1951. He was then the Regius Professor of Physic at Cambridge University and I had submitted a thesis for the Degree of Doctor of Medicine on work I had done in the Pneumoconiosis Research Unit at Cardiff on movement of the chest and diaphragm during respiration.

Cambridge still had a medieval tradition of expecting a candidate for this degree to 'keep an Act'. The candidate was cross questioned about his thesis by the Regius Professor and an Assessor. But notice of the Act was posted on the screens throughout the University and any graduate could turn up to take part in the discussion. The exam was conducted in a gentlemanly way. There were three of us to be examined that day. We attended at the University Department of

Pathology. Here we were ushered into a room and each was handed a slip of paper requesting that we write a short essay on a subject relating to our thesis. (This was to show that we really were the people who had written the theses.) I had written about three pages of my essay when a butler entered with glasses of sherry. So we stopped writing.

When it came my turn (having a name beginning with W, I was of course the last candidate) to enter the examiners' room. I was cross questioned by the Assessor, Dr Cole, while Professor Whitby read my essay. When Dr Cole had finished, Whitby asked me, 'Wade, how do spell paid?' 'P-a-y-e-d,' I said. 'Oh, said Whitby, 'I am not sure that I can give an MD to someone who spells it that way.' He smiled and dismissed me. I have always spelt that word correctly ever since.

Not only was the profusion of new sulphonamide derivatives of immediate value in the treatment of a large variety of infectious diseases but in retrospect it can be seen to have been accompanied by the birth of three important concepts, designing drugs, assessing not only their benefits but also their drawbacks and the role of competitive inhibition. I say birth advisedly for each concept could be said to have had an earlier conception and could perhaps be said to have already been in gestation, yet for all practical purposes, their birth coincided with the introduction of the sulphonamides; all three concepts were to play an important part in the development of pharmacology during my professional life.

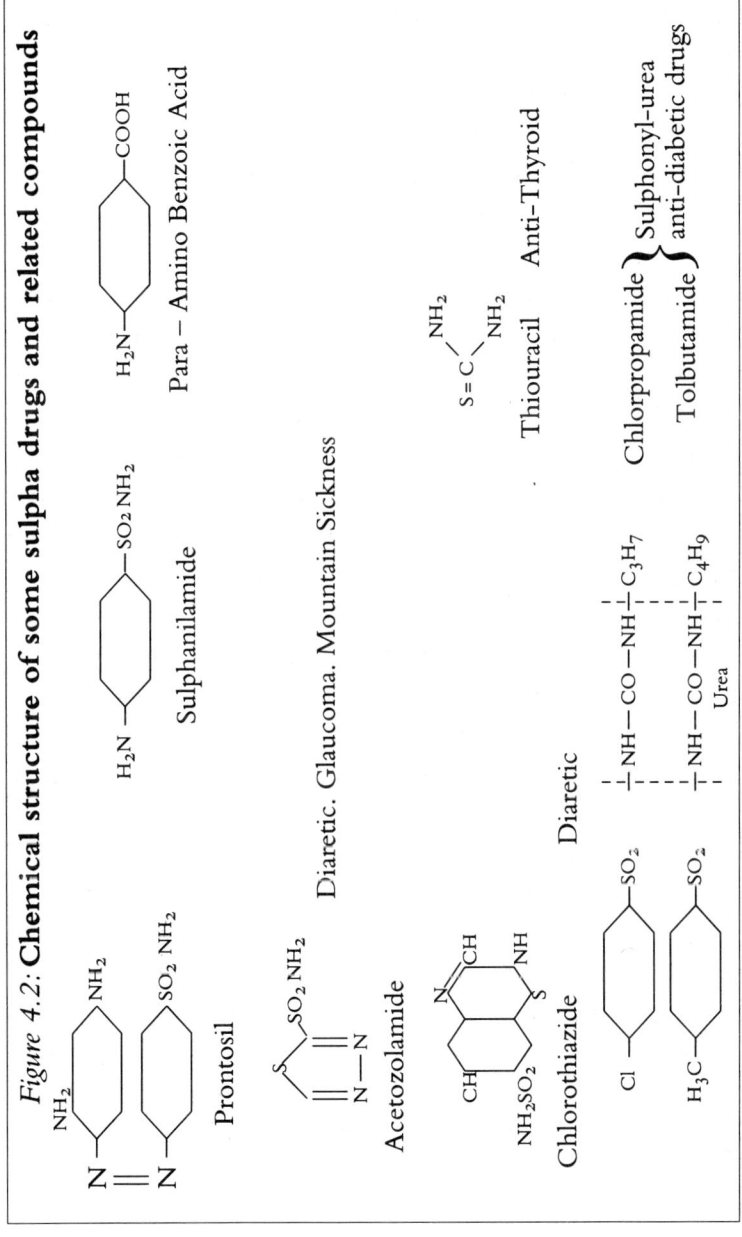

Figure 4.2: **Chemical structure of some sulpha drugs and related compounds**

Designing drugs

It was rapidly shown that different sulphonamide drugs had different properties which could be exploited. Succinylsulphathiazol, sulphaguanidine and phthalylsulphathiazol were shown to be largely unabsorbed in the intestinal tract. They could be used to treat some intestinal infections such as dysentery and were useful in reducing the intestinal content of bacteria before surgery. Sulphacetamide and sulphisoxazole had a high solubility in urine and a low renal toxicity. Other sulphonamides were found to be rapidly absorbed from the gut but slowly excreted in the urine. For the first time the pharmaceutical industry could begin to think about designing new drugs for specific purposes and dreams of exploiting structure/action relationships seemed just a little nearer to reality. Psychologically it was important, for it heralded new thinking and new approaches in drug development.

Benefits versus disadvantages

It was experience with the use of the sulphonamides which first alerted the medical profession to the idea that great benefits might be accompanied by, in some patients, serious adverse reactions. Acute haemolytic anaemia, occasionally agranulocytosis and thrombocytopaenia and rarely aplastic anaemia were all reported in patients receiving sulphonamides. Rashes were common but only rarely was the serious but sometimes fatal Stevens Johnson syndrome seen.

Sulphonamides

When I was appointed to the Chair in Pharmacology and Therapeutics at Queen's University Belfast in 1957, I realised for the first time how common these reactions were, because general practitioners, knowing that the new chair had been created, came to me for help. I was nonplussed; till then I did not realise there was a serious problem.

In 1960 when I was going to the Medical Research Council Headquarters on London to a meeting concerned with a trial of antibiotics in the treatment of bronchitis, I made an appointment to see Sir Harold Himsworth, the then Secretary to the Council, to suggest that a multicentre investigation should be mounted to characterise these adverse reactions.

I remember being slightly disconcerted when I went in to see Himsworth, who had been my Professor of Medicine when I trained at University College Hospital and who knew me quite well. He greeted me and then teased me because I had a small slide rule in my breast-pocket. He wondered what medicine was coming to when professors of medicine went around with slide rules in their pockets. Nowadays, of course, anyone who had ever used a slide rule is looked on, in this computer age, as if he were Neanderthal man!

Himsworth listened to what I had to say about adverse reactions to drugs but it was clear that he felt that I was a young new professor with fire in my belly for this particular project but that the project was not important enough to be taken on board by the Council.

I have wondered since what his reaction would have been two years later in 1962 when the thalidomide disaster first became apparent. It was probably because I had evinced interest and concern about these adverse reaction that I was appointed to the Dunlop Committee when it was created in 1964, although I was far the youngest and most junior member.

Competitive inhibition

The first rational explanation of the mode of action of the sulpha drugs was made by Fildes and Woods. They showed that para-aminobenzoic acid (PABA) is an essential requirement of those bacteria the growth of which is inhibited by the sulphonamides. If present in large concentration the sulpha drugs prevent the bacteria incorporating PABA into pteroylglutamic acid or folic acid, which contains a PABA radical and which is an essential metabolite needed when these bacteria multiply. Sulphanilamide is very similar in its chemical structure to PABA and it competes with PABA for incorporation into the bacteria but cannot be used by the bacteria in the way that PABA is to produce folic acid. Once multiplication of the bacteria is diminished the defence systems of the patient can deal with the infection effectively.

Much of the thinking of those who have since developed beta adrenergic receptor drugs so useful in the control of high blood pressure, or the H_2 blocking drugs that have revolutionised that treatment of peptic ulcers, must have been influenced by this early work on the mode of action of the sulphonamides.

Disappointment

Nothing was more devastating to my contemporaries than the realisation that the sulphonamides were totally ineffective against the tubercle bacillus. This disappointment was recur when it was found that penicillin was also ineffective. We had to await the arrival in 1948 of streptomycin. To my generation this was perhaps the most dramatic of all the new generation of anti-infection drugs, for tuberculosis was so firmly fixed in our minds as 'the captain of the men of death'. It was a little compensation that dapsone, closely related to the sulphonamides, was the first effective drug against leprosy.

The unanticipated and the astonishing

It was to dawn on us slowly that newly synthesised agents may be endowed with unanticipated pharmacological properties; these were usually regarded initially as being unwanted properties; no one foresaw they could lead us to new and exciting developments.

Diuretics

A minor problem in the use of sulphanilamide which was first described in 1937 was that a disturbance of the acid-based equilibrium of the blood might occur;

there was a loss of sodium and potassium in the urine and a decrease in the carbon dioxide combining power of the serum. This acidosis might be accompanied by hyperpnea. There was initially a lot of argument as to why this acidosis occurred; some thought the acidosis was secondary to the hyperventilation, others that it was an alkali-deficit acidosis due to the loss of base in the urine. Then in the early 1950s it was shown that sulphanilamide inhibited the enzyme carbonic anhydrase *in vitro* and, *in vivo* inhibited the normal acidification of urine and caused a minor diuresis. A large number of sulphonamides were synthesised and tested for their ability it inhibit carbonic anhydrase and for their usefulness as diuretics. One of the first drugs to be developed was acetazolamide but within a few years a large number of more potent thiazide diuretics had been synthesised. Chlorothiazide and bendrofluthiazide are still widely used not only as diuretics but also in the treatment of high blood pressure.

Because the enzyme carbonic anhydrase plays an important role in the formation of the aqueous humour of the eye, acetazolamide had been of enormous use in the treatment of glaucoma and in recent years, mainly as a consequence of research carried out under most difficult circumstances by my colleagues in the Birmingham Medical Expeditionary Society in the Himalayas, it had been shown to be most valuable in preventing the onset of high altitude mountain sickness.

Sulphonamides

Antithyroid drugs

In 1941 Julia and Colin Mackenzie and E. V. McCollum working at Johns Hopkins Hospital, Baltimore, were using sulphaguanidine to inhibit gut flora in nutritional studies in animals and observed that the animals developed goitres. A similar observation was made within the next few months by Richter and Clisby with phenylthiourea which was being used for experiments on taste in rats. These two drugs were to be the prototypes of a number of drugs which interfere with the iodinisation of tyrosine and the formation of thyroxine.

One of my first clinical attachments as a medical student in 1943 was to the Medical Unit at University College Hospital where Professor Harold Himsworth was using thiouracil for the first time in the UK for the treatment of hyperthyroidism. I can remember clearly, despite the burden of air raid casualties that our Hospital was bearing in war-torn London, how exciting it was to have a medical treatment for a disease, for which at that time only surgery and partial thyroidectomy was available, which in ill wasted patients was, with the anaesthesia available in those days, always hazardous.

Antidiabetic drugs

It was in France suffering from overwhelming German defeat that, in 1942 at Montpellier, Janbon and coworkers, trying unsuccessfully to find whether sulphonamides were of any value in typhoid fever, first showed that the sulpha drug might induce hypoglycaemia. Not

75

surprisingly this observation was not followed up until after the war. A number of sulphonylurea compounds were then examined for hypoglycaemic properties which were shown to be caused by an increased release of insulin from the beta cells of the pancreas. Thus tolbutamide and chlorpropamide were developed as valuable drugs in the treatment of late onset non-insulin dependent diabetes.

Conclusion

It is not surprising that I look back on the sulphonamides with some nostalgia. My father's life was save by them in 1936 and they and their derivatives have been bound into and entwined with my professional career. The lessons that have been learnt from them are part of modern pharmacology.

CHAPTER 5

Penicillin

Penicillin was discovered and many of its properties known long before Domagk started to work on the sulphonamides but it only became available for clinical use in 1942 and only properly available in 1943 and 1944. I was privileged to see its introduction when I was a student and a house-officer at University College Hospital, London from 1942 to 1947 and I have also been privileged to know personally many who played important parts in its discovery and development, which although so frequently described still fascinates and astonishes me.

St Mary's Hospital

Almroth Wright was the son of a vicar. His mother was a Swede. He was schooled in Belfast and he took an honours degree at Trinity College, Dublin before he took up medicine. After graduation he worked with Cohnheim in Leipzig before he was appointed as the Professor of Pathology at the Army School of Medicine at Netley. It was he who developed a vaccine made from killed typhoid bacilli which protected 14,000 of the 330,000 British troops who took part in the Boer war, and would have protected many more but for

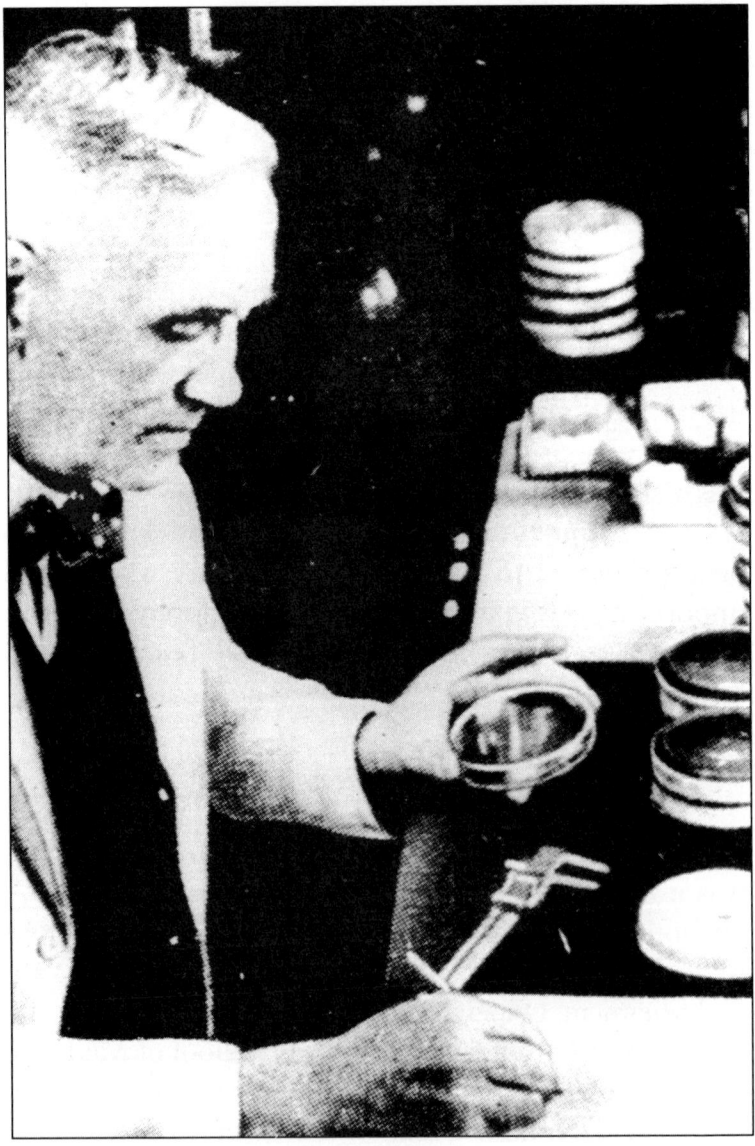

Figure 5.1: Dr Fleming working at St Mary's hospital, London

opposition to its use; officers actually threw the vaccine overboard because troops disliked the initial but short lived discomfort and fever that followed its administration. In 1902 Wright became Professor of Bacteriology and Pathology at St Mary's Hospital and six years later was able to found a separate and independent Inoculation Department of which he was the Director. He was a rude, uncouth, energetic and enthusiastic man and he believed in immunity as only a believer can believe.

Alexander Fleming, a dour Scot, joined Wright in 1905. He was very welcome at St Mary's as a valuable member of the rifle team. In 1922 with very little encouragement from Wright, Fleming began to look at the protective properties of mucus and tears and he showed that a constituent which he called lysozyme was bactericidal. The work that he did on lysozyme seems to me to almost a 'trailer' for the big film on penicillin because:

Fleming's interest in it was aroused by a contaminated culture plate.

He immediately recognised the significance of the substance.

His enthusiasm had a cool reception from his colleagues, especially Wright.

He worked on it with dogged determination and patience.

He was thwarted because no chemist could extract
and characterise the active material.

The discovery of penicillin

In 1928 the observation of a culture plate contaminated
with a mould, *Penicillium notatum*, which had inhibited
bacterial growth led Fleming to determine the antibacterial properties of penicillin. He showed that it had
bactericidal properties against staphylococci, streptococci, cornybacteria that caused diphtheria, clostridia,
meningococci and pneumococci when these bacteria
were growing in culture media. Its potential for the
treatment of the many common and life threatening
infections of mankind was obvious. But the task of
isolating, purifying and characterising the active material was beyond the resources of those times: Ridley
tried at St Mary's in 1929 and Raistrick at the London
School of Tropical Medicine and Hygiene in 1932.

The first known attempt to use penicillin to treat an
infection in man was by Fleming. He washed out the
infect nasal sinuses of a colleague, Stuart Craddock,
in 1929; but the solution he used probably contained
very little penicillin and it is doubtful whether it was
of any value as treatment. More effective, but poorly
recorded, was the use in 1930 and 1931 of topical
preparations of crude penicillin by C. G. Paine,
Lecturer in Bacteriology at Sheffield, to treat conjunc-
tival infections. There was a better recorded successful

treatment of a patient with pneumococcal conjuncti-
vities by K. B. Rogers at St Mary's.

The development at Oxford

Howard Florey came from Adelaide to the Chair in
Pathology in Sheffield in 1932. He learnt of Paine's
work and when he went to Oxford in 1934 he encour-
aged the chemist Ernst Chain, a refugee from Nazi
Germany, to work on lysozyme and penicillin. In late
1939 or early 1940 Chain obtained penicillin in a pretty
murky solution and by freeze drying he was able to
concentrate it as a crude yellow powder. There was
just enough of this crude preparation for it to be tried
out on the 20 May 1940 in three groups of mice infected
with different organisms; the experiment was carried
out by Norman Heatley who sat up all night recording
the results of the experiment. It was on that day that
Guderian's panzer Corps reached the sea at Abbeville,
and, but for Hitler's perverse order to the Corps to
halt, it would have decimated the British Expeditionary
Force which over the next few days escaped from
Dunkirk.

A further experiment was carried out on the 1 July
1940 and the work was reported in the *Lancet* of 24
August. It was only after the publication of this paper
that Ernst Chain discovered that Alex Fleming was still
alive! Desperate efforts were then made to culture
Penicillium notatum to obtain more penicillin. Stacks of

bedpans were filled with culture media and the *Penicillium notatum* grown on the surface of the media.

By January 1941 there was enough penicillin available for Florey to approach Leslie Witts, the Professor of Medicine at Oxford to ask for help. Florey explained that although penicillin appeared to be harmless to leucocytes, tissue cultures and many different laboratory animal species, he was apprehensive of giving the first injection to a healthy volunteer in case some unpleasant reaction might occur. It was Charles Fletcher, in the presence of Florey and Witts, who gave the first injection to a human being. It was 17 January 1941. The patient was Mrs Elva Akers. She was a 50-year-old woman who was dying of disseminated breast cancer. She agreed to take part in this experiment. She knew why it was being done and she knew that it would not do her any good and she accepted that she might suffer some unforeseen unpleasant reaction.

Fortunately it caused this courageous woman no other trouble than a rigor and a transient fever; it was one of the problems with many of the early impure preparations of penicillin that they contained pyrogens. It was encouraging that a blood sample taken from Mrs Akers a few hours later was shown by the microbiologists to have a high enough concentration of penicillin to be bactericidal.

Early clinical use at Oxford in 1941

The first patient to be treated with penicillin was a

policeman aged 43; he had been ill for four months with staphylococcal and streptococcal septicaemia and multiple abscess in his lungs and on his face and he had osteomyelitis of the right humerus. Penicillin was started on 12 February; 10,000 units (200 mg) was given intravenously through an in-dwelling needle (cannulas were not everyday equipment then as now!) and followed every three hours with 15,000 units. The treatment was continued for five days. The patient made a dramatic improvement. But there was no more penicillin with which to continue treatment and his condition deteriorated and he died a month later.

Five more patients were treated; a boy with a wound infected by streptococci, a man with a huge staphylococcal carbuncle which resolved dramatically within five days, a boy aged 4½ years, who had a septic thrombosis in the cavernous sinus, part of the venous drainage system of the brain, in whom the infection was cured but who died due to rupture of a mycotic aneurysm of the carotid artery and another boy of 14 years with osteomyelitis and bacteraemia who was given 860,000 units a day for two weeks and was completely cured – a miracle for all who had seen the indolent chronic and often fatal course that was to be expected in such patients at that time.

It was only a tiny series of clinical cases but it was enough. Florey and Heatley were flown over the USA to persuade the American pharmaceutical industry to do what, under the constraints of war conditions, could not be done in our country, to develop the large scale production of penicillin. This was also attempted at Nestlé's cheese factory at Aylesbury and Glaxo's pharmaceutical factory at Greenford. But the credit for the rapid commercial production of penicillin must go to the American pharmaceutical industry.

Strangely the next year, 1942, Ernst Chain was admitted with a chest infection to the ward on which I was a clinical student at University College Hospital, London. I had to take his clinical history and he told me that he had been a refugee from Nazi Germany and was a chemist, but I did not know anything about his work with penicillin. I do know however that he was not treated with penicillin for at that time we had none. In 1948 just before he went to Rome as the Director of the newly created International Centre for Chemical Microbiology, Dr Chain married his co-worker, Anne Beloff, who had been a fellow student of my wife.

Penicillin becomes available

By early 1943 limited supplies of penicillin were becoming available to hospitals in the United Kingdom. Very wisely the Ministry of Supply had anticipated the difficulties which would arise and had created a General Penicillin Committee in September 1942. The limited supply was allocated in such a way that the value of the antibiotic would be competently assessed in such varied condition as osteomyelitis, mastoid infections, meningitis, venereal disease and sub-acute bacterial endocarditis. The treatment of this last condition was

under the supervision of Ronald Christie, Professor of
Medicine at St Batholemew's Hospital and I remember
the elan and excitement when these patients were seen
to be recovering and their infection cured. It was amazing. It had never been seen before. No elaborate controlled clinical trials were needed to show how effective
penicillin was. It still amazes me, especially as the doses
of penicillin administered were by today's standards
minute; 8,000–12,000 units three times a day!

It was a wonderful time. Even for a young person
like me it was wonderful and for doctors who for years
had been able to do so little for patients with conditions
such as bacterial endocarditis it was unbelievable.

It was in 1948 when I joined the staff of the Pneumokoniosis Research Unit of the Medical Research
Council at Cardiff that I first met Charles Fletcher. He
was the Director of the Unit. He was a modest man
and he never spoke about his work at Oxford; I did
not learn of his part in the development of penicillin
till many years later.

In 1964 after the thalidomide disaster, I was to work
closely with Leslie Witts. We were both appointed as
members of the Committee on Safety of Drugs, the
'Dunlop Committee'. He was Chairman and I Vice-
Chairman of the Adverse Reactions Sub-Committee.
By that time I did of course know of the part that he
had played at Oxford and on several occasions we
discussed the extraordinary good fortune that penicillin,
besides being so effective an antibiotic, was so remark-
ably free of adverse reactions.

The Romance of Remedies

The first use of penicillin in war casualties

When I went to work at Cardiff in 1948 near neigh-
bours, with whom Margaret and I made great friends,
were Scott and Dorothy Thomson. Their children were
the same age as ours. Scott was the Head of the Public
Health Laboratory Service at Cardiff and was later to
be appointed the Professor of Bacteriology at the Welsh
School of Medicine. I was much interested in his work
and I think I might quite easily have joined Scott and
become a microbiologist.

I have a photograph of Scott in uniform taken at
Oxford in March 1943 when he and Dorothy were
married at rather short notice because he was being
sent out to North Africa. He had been called to Oxford
for a crash course of two weeks on penicillin with Forey
before he and a young surgeon, Ian Fraser, later to be
a senior colleague of mine at the Royal Victoria Hospital Belfast, were sent to North Africa to conduct the
first trials of penicillin on war casualties in the forward
area.

They saw the drug being produced, were taught how
to use it and advised how to organise a mobile laboratory in a forward area. They were very impressed.
Florey had turned his laboratory almost into a factory.
The penicillin they produced and gave to patients contained a lot of contaminants from the culture medium
on which the *Penicillium* was grown. It was a brown
powder and in solution it looked like dilute mustard,
and when injected it felt just like that.

Professor Florey's wife, Ethel, was busy every day on

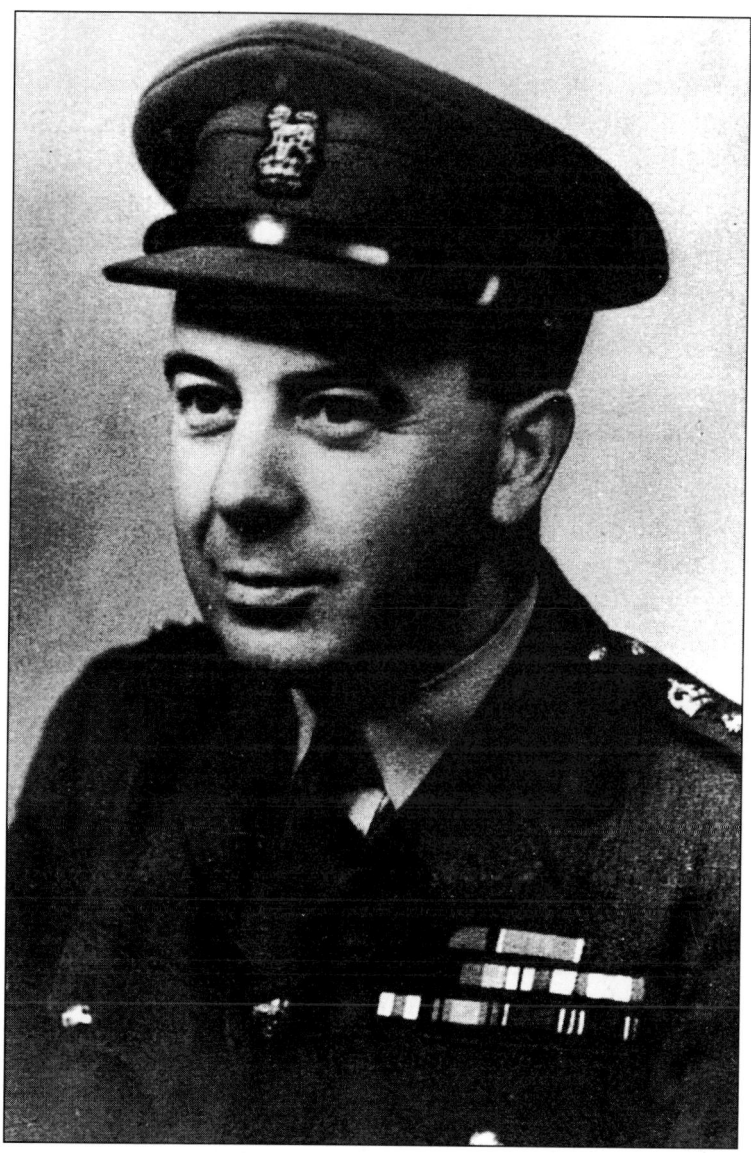

Figure 5.2: Mr Ian Fraser

her bicycle collecting the overnight urine of all patients on penicillin in the Oxford hospitals. This urine was valuable. It contained about 2/3rds of the penicillin that had been given to the patients and about half of it could be retrieved. Moreover it was free of the contaminants from the culture medium and injection of it was painless so that it was very popular.

The African and Italian experience

Thomson and Fraser sailed to Algiers on a small hospital ship, the *Newfoundland*, which was later sunk. The work in Algiers was disappointing for the patients there were all suffering from long standing sepsis. They understood why Florey had had to say to doctors in Oxford, 'Send my you patients early. I cannot resurrect a corpse.'

Fortunately, the invasion of Sicily was imminent. Fraser embarked on the hospital carrier *St David*; before the war she ran the packet service between Fishguard and Rosslare. He landed near Cape Passero to send casualties back to the *St David*. It was mighty hectic. They operated continuously on severe casualties. Forty-six operations were done in fifty-four hours. When they left they had 154 patients on the ship of which 5 died. As usual when fighting is at close quarters most of the injuries were bullet wounds, 73% to limbs, 22% to the body and trunk and 5% to the head and neck.

He made a second visit on 27 July with another surgeon, Jim Jeffery. The results with penicillin were

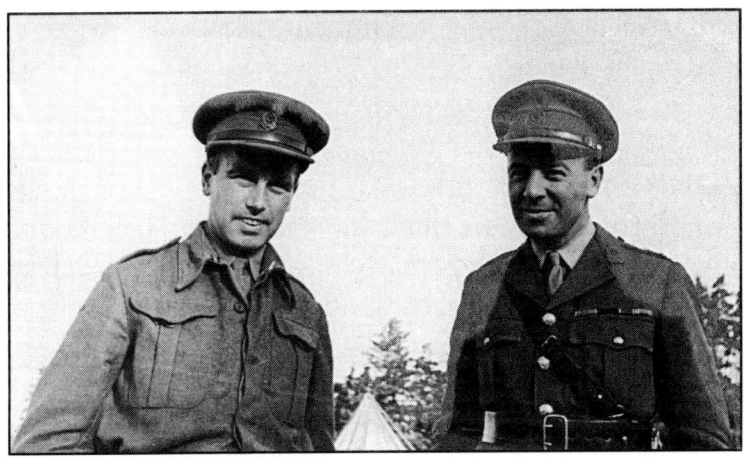

Figure 5.2: Dr Scott Thomson and Mr Ian Fraser who supervised the first use of penicillin in war casualties in Sicily and Italy.

magnificent. Patients arrived at forward base hospitals with clean wounds ready for definitive surgery. Pon D'abreu, an experienced surgeon who had worked with my father in Cardiff before the war and with whom I was later to work in Birmingham, sent a signal to Fraser, 'What the hell are you doing? We have never seen the like of this before.'

After Sicily was conquered, Italy was invaded. Then a landing was made much further north on the west Italian coast at Salerno. Here the landing was resisted not by Italians who were fed up with the war, but by the Germans. The struggle was long and difficult but before it had finished Fraser went down with diphtheria and was evacuated to Cairo. Jeffery and Scott Thomson continued the work but the saga was over. Treatment with penicillin became a routine rather than a piece of experimental research.

Conclusion

I was fortunate. I saw medicine and surgery before and after penicillin. In those early days it was unbelievable. What made us most sad was that penicillin was of no value in treating tuberculosis. This was a disappointment soon to be forgotten, when streptomycin became available in 1948 and para-aminobenzoic acid in 1951.

CHAPTER 6

Streptomycin

When I was a medical student in 1942 tuberculosis was still one the 'captains of the men of death'. In the UK with improvement in housing and nutrition the mortality had fallen from 250 per 1000 at the beginning of the century to 49. 5 per 1000 in the 1940s.

Medical students, doctors and nurses were at greater risk than the rest of the community. Of the sixty students in my clinical year at University College Hospital, London in 1942 three developed tuberculosis and were sent to sanatoria. One came back to finish her training.

In our wards tuberculosis was common and the first patient that I clerked when I had finished my introductory clinical course and started on a medical ward, had pulmonary tuberculosis. I remember Kitty well. Her parents ran a small Italian restaurant in Euston Road.

Three years later in 1945 when I had qualified and was working as a house-officer on the same ward, she was readmitted and died. I wrote to her family doctor, Dr Ripka of Gower Street. He wrote back a letter which I have kept because I appreciated it so much.

I very much liked Kitty and with her memory in mind I will always think of your moving remarks that you were very sorry to see Kitty die, that she

91

was an old friend and was the first patient you had ever clerked as a student and that you wished you had been able to do more for her. Your kind words will be a great source of consolation to the relatives when I show them your letter.

Tuberculosis was only too common in young adults at that time. In the paediatric wards I saw children dying of tuberculous meningitis for which there was no effective treatment, for once the diagnosis was made death was inevitable.

The great disappointment when I was a student was that neither the sulphonamides nor penicillin were of any use in the treatment of tuberculosis.

Streptomycin

Did I but know it, but even as I was watching Kitty die work was already in hand that was going to bring new hope to all who suffered from tuberculosis.

On 1 June 1943 the National Tuberculosis Association of the USA had called a meeting at the Pennsylvania Hotel, New York, of interested parties to discuss, in the light of the recent successful development of penicillin, the possibility of developing a chemotherapeutic agent effective against the *Mycobacterium tuberculosis.*

One of those who attended that meeting was Selman Wakesman. He was a microbiologist working at an Agricultural Research Station in New Jersey. Since 1916 he had been studying the microbiological population of soils particularly the various saprophytes. In

Streptomycin

1940 he had isolated actinomycin, a red pigmented compound highly active in destroying various bacteria but extremely toxic when administers to animals. (A closely related compound was later shown to be of value as a cytotoxic agent in the treatment of cancer.)

In 1942 he had isolated another compound, streptothricin. This was also active against many common pathogenic bacteria but it was also very toxic when injected into animals. Possibly for this reason its effects of *Mycobacterium tuberculosis* were not tested until after the 1943 New York meeting. It was shown that it was active against that organism.

But within a year a new compound was isolated which looked much more promising. One day in early August 1943 a New Jersey farmer observed one of his chickens was ill with breathing trouble. Fearing an epidemic at his poultry farm he took the animal to the Agricultural Experimental Station. The pathologist took a swab of the chicken's throat. This was cultured and three colonies of actinomyces were observed.

These were shown to Dr Wakesman and on 20 August 1943 he identified the organism as identical with one which he and his colleague Dr Curtis had isolated from soil and identified in 1916. Then it had been called *Actinomyces griseum* but the generic name had since been changed and it was now called *Streptomyces griseum*. It was soon shown that it produced a compound, Streptomycin, that was extremely effective against *Mycobacterium tuberculosis*.

93

William Feldman and H. Corner Hinshaw of the
Mayo Clinic, Rochester, using a crude preparation of
Wakesman's streptomycin, carried out some promising
preliminary studies in guinea pigs that were completed
by July 1944. Further more extensive animal studies
soon confirmed this work. Although Feldman and Hinshaw were enthusiastic about the effectiveness of streptomycin in the treatment of experimental tuberculosis
in animals, they were rightly very restrained in the
claims they made in their published work.

By this time more and purer streptomycin was available and it was decided that the first clinical trial of
streptomycin in patients with tuberculosis was justified.
This took place at the Mayo clinic in the winter of
1944–5.

Here is the report of the first patient treated with
streptomycin.

November 20th 1944 was the day on which streptomycin was first administered to a human being
for the treatment of tuberculosis. The patient was
a 21-year-old white girl who had progressive far
advanced tuberculosis . . . When she was admitted
to the Sanatorium in July 1943 this patient had
advanced pulmonary tuberculosis involving the
right upper lobe.

During her first year of hospitalization she
showed some improvement, but shortly afterwards
she began to have chills, fever, night sweats and
increased cough; a chest roentgenogram obtained
in October 1944 showed a pronounced increased

in infiltration and cavitation in the right lung . . .
At this point it was decided that the patient's pro-
gressively unfavourable course made the use of
streptomycin justifiable and desirable.

Accordingly some of the material then being used
in the guinea pig experiment was appropriated for
this first clinical trial. As the therapeutic and toxic
doses of streptomycin for human beings were entirely unknown, the drug was administered with
extreme caution. At first the total daily dose was
only o. 1 Gm and this amount was divided into
eight doses given at three-hour intervals around the
clock. From the first the drug was given by deep
intramuscular injection.

The first preparations of streptomycin were relatively crude . . . Between November 20th, 1944,
and April 7th, 1945, the patient received five courses
of streptomycin, each of which lasted ten to eight-
een days. The treatment was interrupted partly to
give relief from side effects but mostly because at
that time a steady supply of streptomycin was not
available.

This patient was discharged from the sanatorium
on July 13, 1947, with a diagnosis of apparently
arrested pulmonary tuberculosis. There was no
deterioration of her condition as revealed by peri-
odic examinations. She had since married and is
the mother of three children, born in 1950, 1952
and 1954.

Not all patients were as fortunate as that young lady.

The clinical results at the Mayo Clinic were encouraging but were by no means conclusive. The natural course of pulmonary tuberculosis is so variable and unpredictable that evidence of improvement or cure in a few cases following the use of a new drug could not be accepted as proof of its effectiveness. Physicians remembered only too well the enthusiastic introduction of the gold salt, sodium aurothiosulphate, in 1924. It had been shown to be effective in killing *Mycobacterium tuberculosis* in culture in the laboratory. And after an optimistic report of its effectiveness in the treatment of patients with tuberculosis by Dr Möllgard in Copenhagen, it was accepted uncritically by the medical profession. Its rapid reception and wide use was followed by disappointment and, after ten years, complete rejection for there was no firm evidence of benefit from its use and it caused unpleasant skin rashes and renal damage.

First use of streptomycin in Britain

In the UK streptomycin first became available in very small amounts in late 1946. The Medical Research Council decided that the small supply of streptomycin given to it for research purposes would best be employed in a rigorously planned investigation with concurrent controls. A Tuberculosis Trials Committee was set up under the Chairmanship of Geoffrey Marshall. One of the members of the Committee was a statistician, Professor Austin Bradford Hill, and his hand can be seen in the planning of this and the two subsequent controlled clinical trails of streptomycin.

One of the centres at which these trials were carried out was Sully Hospital near Cardiff, where my eldest brother was a thoracic surgeon. I was working in the Medical Research Council's Pneumoconiosis Research Unit at Llandough Hospital about five miles from Sully. I knew Mr Dillwyn Thomas and the Australian physician, Dr Leonard West, who were responsible for the work at Sully well and I remember how exciting this work was for all of us.

The plan

It was decided that only young patients aged 15 to 25 years old (later extended to 30) with acute progressive bilateral pulmonary tuberculosis of recent origin and bacteriologically proven would be included in the trial. All patients would be admitted to hospital and treated with complete bed rest, but half of them would be allocated randomly to receive streptomycin 2 grams daily.

Assessment was based on changes in the X-ray pictures, weight, temperature, sedimentation rate and bacillary content of the sputum. The most important assessments were the X-ray changes. All radiographs were viewed by an independent panel of two radiologists and a clinician who played no part in the treatment of the patients in the trial and who did not know which patients were receiving streptomycin.

The results

At the end of six months of treatment 4 of the 55 streptomycin patients had died. Of the 52 control patients who had not received streptomycin 14 had died. The probability of this difference occurring by chance was less than 1 in 100.

The radiological assessments of the patients after six months were:

	Streptomycin	Control
Considerable improvement	28	4
Moderate improvement	10	13
No change	2	3
Moderate deterioration	5	12
Considerable deterioration	6	6
Death	4	14

There was also substantially more improvement in the weight, temperature, sedimentation rate, and bacillary count in the sputum in the patients receiving streptomycin compared with those who did not receive it.

In many of the patients who received streptomycin and did not improve it was found that the tubercle bacilli had become resistant to streptomycin. Another

---

Opposite: Figure 6.1
The results of three Medical Research Council clinical trials of the treatment of pulmonary tuberculosis with bed rest, streptomycin and PAS and streptomycin. (After Daniels, M. and Hill, A.B.. *Brit. med. Journal* (1952) 1. 1162.)

Streptomycin

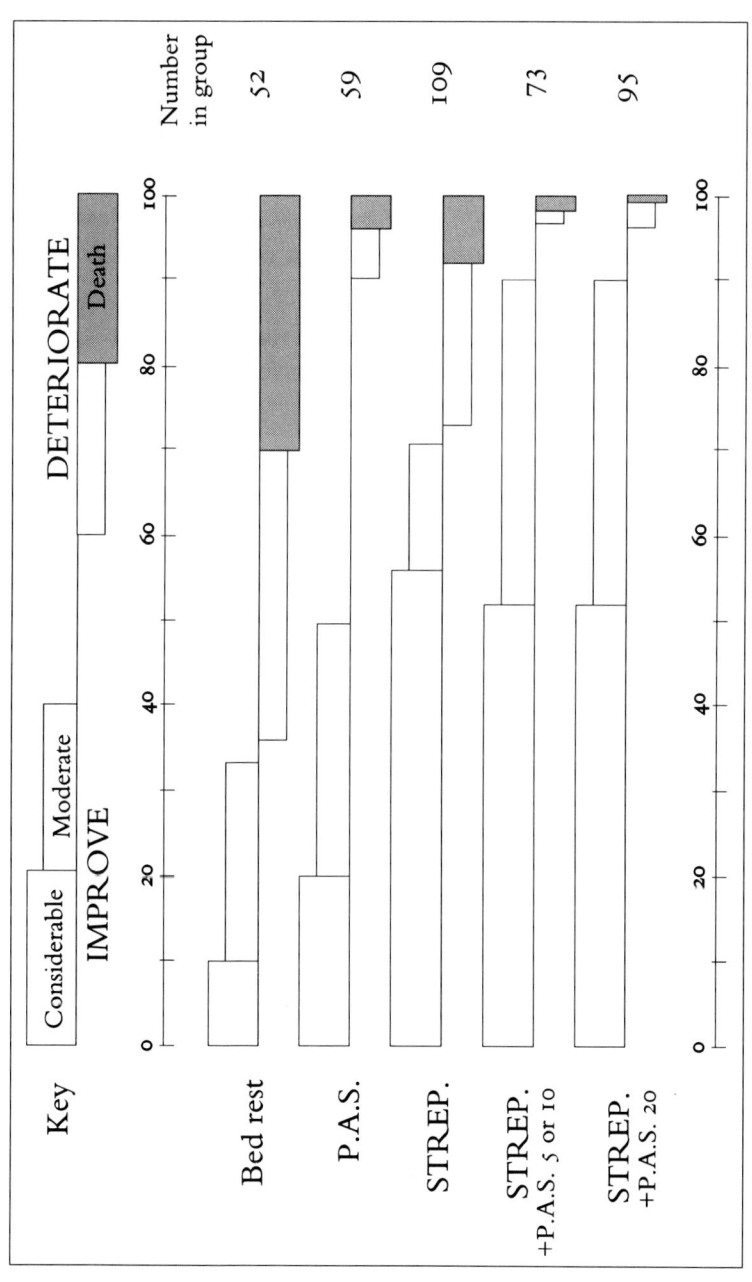

problem, which had been anticipated, was that many of the patients receiving streptomycin suffered toxic damage to the auditory and vestibular system with deafness and balance difficulty.

In 1948 another drug effective against *Mycobacterium tuberculosis* was discovered, para-aminosalicylic acid (PAS). Two years later a second trial was arranged to compare the effects of daily administration of 1 gram streptomycin alone, (1 gram instead of 2 gram to reduce the incidence of vestibular and auditory damage), 20 grams of PAS alone and the two drugs together.

It was clearly shown in this trial that when the two drugs were taken together there was a substantial reduction in the development of streptomycin resistant organisms. However the large doses of PAS produced nausea and vomiting in so many patients that a third trial was set up in which 1 gram of streptomycin a day was given with 20 grams, 10 gram and 5 gram of PAS.

What made this series of clinical trials so impressive was that all the patients admitted to the three trials were so similar – young aged 15–30, with acute progressive bilateral bacteriologically proven pulmonary tuberculosis unsuitable for collapse therapy. All patients were randomly allocated to the treatment regimens and all were assessed according to a plan agreed before the first trial in 1946.

There was a link deliberately planned between the successive trials. The first and second trials each had a group treated with streptomycin alone. The second and third trials each had a group treated with streptomycin and 20 gram of PAS each day. The overlap of a similarly treated group from one trial to the next was there to show that it was fair to make comparisons between the differently treated patients in all three trials. In particular it allowed comparison of patients in the second and third trial to be compared with the patients in the first trial, who were not treated with either of the drugs. It would have been ethically unjustified to include again such a group of patients who had no chemotherapy. The inclusion of such a group was justifiable in 1947 when there was so little streptomycin available and there were still doubts about its efficacy in the treatment of tuberculosis.

Conclusion

This was a wonderful piece of work. The comprehensive planning and analysis of the three relatively small 'controlled clinical trials' became a model for the assessment of new drugs. It influenced British medical practice profoundly and many years later when I visited the American Food and Drugs Administration in Washington, the practice of the British Committee on Safety of Drugs of accepting as proof of the efficacy of a new drug only the results of properly conducted and properly 'controlled' clinical trials was spoken of with awe and envy.

It influenced me greatly. I had the unforgettable experience, available to very few people, of close association with Dillwyn Thomas and Len West in the MRC trials of streptomycin at Sully.

And in the Pneumokoniosis Research Unit I worked with Peter Oldham, a young statistician trained by Bradford Hill, and with Archie Cochrane. Archie's philosophy about 'randomised controlled trials', to be set out so clearly years later in his 1971 Rock Carling publication 'Effectiveness and efficiency', influenced my own work in clinical pharmacology profoundly for the next thirty-odd years of my professional life. I was very lucky and I am very grateful that I had such a wonderful experience.

CHAPTER 7

Thalidomide

The hypnotic which woke us up

Sleep is one of the great balms of life. Sleeplessness due to discomfort or anxiety a great burden and relief from sleeplessness something for which patients seek the help of doctors.

Chloral hydrate is a chlorinated derivative of ethyl alcohol and was first made in 1832 by the great German chemist, Liebig. It was first used as a soporific or hypnotic to encourage sleep in 1869 as an alternative to alcohol or opium, but the first widely used hypnotics were the barbiturates. The first of these was a malonyl-urea compound, sodium barbital, which was marketed in 1903 under a trade name Veronal.

By the time I qualified in 1944 there were at least twenty barbiturate drugs being marketed. Most of them were hypnotic drugs taken by mouth but phenobarbitone was mainly used to control epilepsy and thiopentone was used as an intravenous anaesthetic agent.

One of the problems of the barbiturate hypnotics was that overdose, taken either accidentally, usually by children of toddler age mistaking mummie's tablets for sweeties, or by depressed people wishing to commit suicide, caused respiratory depression which might be fatal.

The other problem was that doctors often found it difficult to withdraw these hypnotics from patients who became dependent on them and continued to take their nightly dose year after year.

It was not surprising therefore that a number of non-barbiturate hypnotic and sedative drugs which were claimed to be less likely to cause respiratory depression and to be lacking in addictive liability gained instant and widespread acceptance. One of the first of these was glutethamide which was marketed in the early 1950s. However despite the claims it was soon found to have many of the disadvantages of the barbiturates. Much more impressive was thalidomide.

Thalidomide

Thalidomide was first marketed in 1956 by the German firm Chemi Grüenthal as Contergan. There was good evidence that even in large overdose it did not produce severe respiratory depression. In Western Europe it was soon widely used under a number of proprietary names and it was often combined with analgesics in tablets for the treatment of pain and cough as well as sleeplessness. These preparations were skilfully promoted and were widely prescribed by doctors. In Germany these preparations could be brought over the counter by the public without a doctor's prescription.

In Britain thalidomide was first marketed in 1958 as

Distaval by Distillers Ltd, a firm of whisky manufacturers which had not had any previous experience in marketing drugs. In Britain its use was much more restricted than on the Continent and it could not be obtained without a doctor's prescription. It was widely promoted to doctors and I have a copy of the *British Medical Journal* of 21 November 1961 with a full page advertisement for Distaval which emphasised its safety and concluded, 'there is no case on record in which even gross overdosage with Distaval has had harmful results. Put you mind at rest. Depend on the safety of Distaval'.

Even then this advertisement was, I thought, economical with the truth because since 1960 there had been several reports associating its use with peripheral neuritis. Patients taking it found the tips of their fingers or their toes were numb. And in September 1961 Dr Pamela Fullerton and Michael Kremer of the Middlesex Hospital had reported in the *British Medical Journal* on thirteen patients who had developed peripheral neuritis while taking the drug, some of them with wasting and weakness of muscles which remained after treatment with the drug had ceased. Worse was soon to follow.

The thalidomide disaster

At a conference of gynaecologists at Kiel on the 19th and 20 October 1961 attention was drawn to the large number of children that had been born in the previous ten months with absent or deformed limbs. Such deformities had previously been rare and concern was expressed that some exogenous cause might have begun to operate. It was suggested that the cause might be one of the many new drugs which were being marketed at that time.

It was Dr Lenz, at a paediatric meeting in Dusseldorf on 19 November 1961, who first suggested that Contergan, a proprietary form of the drug thalidomide might be the responsible agent. There were immediate consultations between medical authorities and Chemi Grüenthal who manufactured thalidomide and the drug was withdrawn from the German market on 25 November 1961.

Investigation soon confirmed Dr Lenz's suspicion. In a survey of ten large obstetric units in Germany it was found that in the ten years to 1959 no children with limb deformities were born; there were 10 in 1959, 26 in 1960 and 477 in 1961.

In another study of 46 mothers delivered of deformed babies, 41 were known to have taken a thalidomide preparation during pregnancy while in a control series of 300 mother delivered of normal babies, none had taken such preparations.

It is now estimated that 6,000 deformed babies were born in West Germany as a result of the use of thalidomide. In Britain there were at least 500 live births of deformed children, some of them dreadfully disabled. This disaster left its mark not only on the children but also on the medical profession, the pharmaceutical

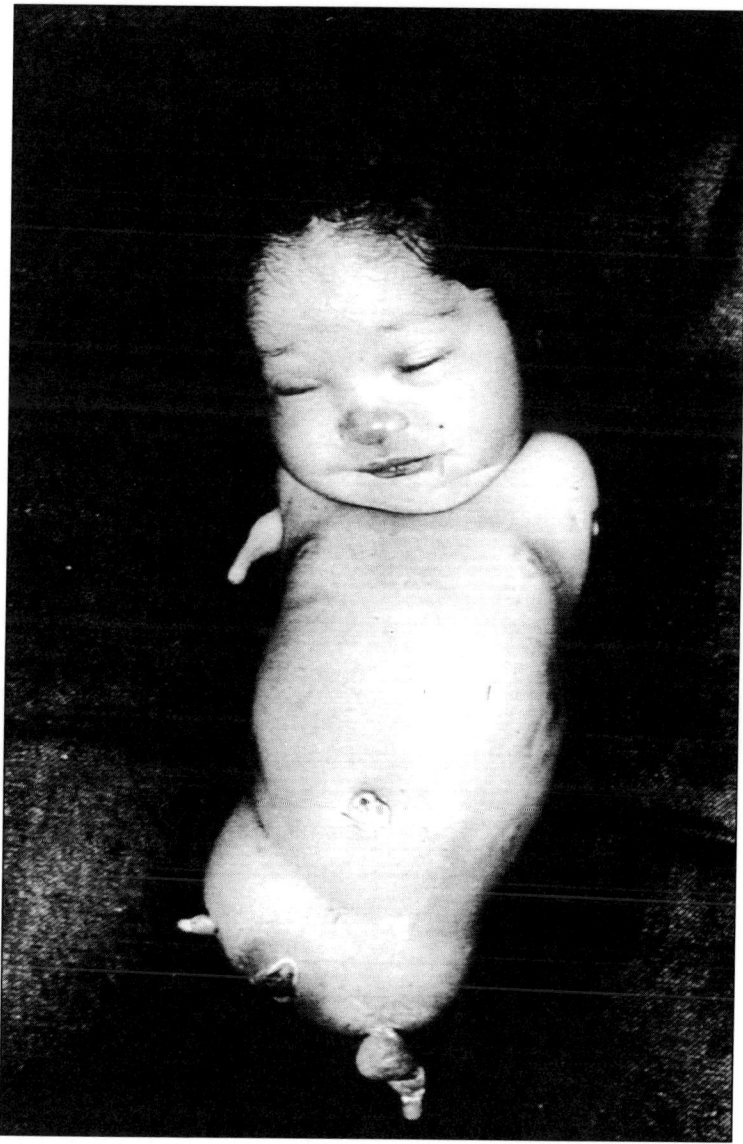

Figure 7.1: This child was born in Belfast with phocomelia. The mother had taken thalidomide early in her pregnancy.

industry and the public. Inevitably, the attention of politicians became focused on the problems of adverse reactions to drugs and this led to the establishment of drug regulatory bodies in many countries throughout the world.

In Britain it led to the creation of the Committee on Safety of Drugs (CSD) in 1963. The Chairman was Professor Derrick Dunlop and much to my surprise, for I was still very young, I was asked to serve on the Committee. I also served as Vice-Chairman under my colleague Leslie Witts on the Adverse Reaction Sub-committee of the CSD. It was work which I was to continue till the end of my professional life.

Early studies in Northern Ireland

When we first learnt of the thalidomide disaster my colleague at Queen's University, Peter Elmes immediately suggested to me that I might ask the Northern Ireland General Health Services Board, NIGHSB, if it could give us any information of the prescribing of thalidomide in Northern Ireland.

I found that the Board had, since the early 1950s, a system of recording and paying for every medicine supplied by pharmacists for the prescriptions written by doctors in general practice in the National Health Service in Northern Ireland.

The system used in Northern Ireland was far more advanced and comprehensive than the system used in England at that time. In England pharmacies sent all the prescription forms they had dealt with each month to the Prescription Pricing Authority in Newcastle on Tyne. There a one in ten sample of the prescriptions was examined and priced manually by trained girls so that the pharmacists could be reimbursed for the medicines they had supplied.

In Northern Ireland there was a large number of small pharmacies. The population of 1½ million people was served by about 750 general practitioners and about 700 pharmacies. As a result the number of prescription forms received by the pricing bureau of the NIGHSB from each pharmacy was so small that if only a one in ten sample had been taken for pricing, a pharmacist might have been grossly overpaid or underpaid for the drugs he had supplied.

For this reason the Board had in 1953 mechanised the pricing system so that all prescriptions written by the general practitioners were priced. The details of every prescription were punched on to Hollerith cards. These are cards with a large number of holes punched around their sides which can be mechanically sorted in such a way that the costs of the preparations supplied by a pharmacist could be quickly and easily ascertained and the pharmacist reimbursed promptly.

Unfortunately when I went to see the Board in January or February 1962 the Hollerith cards and the prescription forms for the months prior to November 1961 had already been destroyed so that I was not able to execute my plan to ascertain which mothers had been prescribed thalidomide during their pregnancy

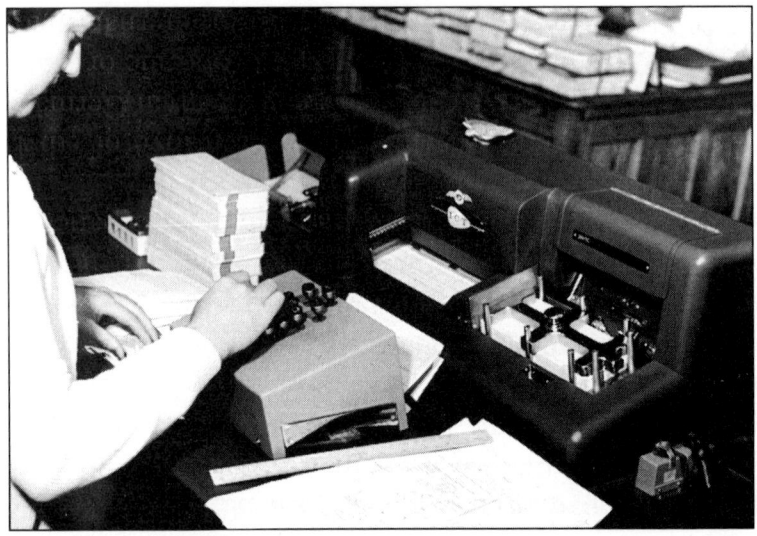

Figure 7.2: Sorting Hollerith cards at the Northern Ireland General Health Services Board in 1962.

and how many had had normal children and how many abnormal children.

I realised however that the Board had a unique system which would allow me to examine in detail the prescribing of every doctor in Northern Ireland and which might make it possible to assess how often rare but serious adverse reactions to an individual drug occurred.

I proceeded with great circumspection because I realised that I would be in danger of arousing the hostility of general practitioners if they felt that they were being spied upon. I discussed the matter with Dr Hunter, the Board's medical officer, and we decided that it would be fully justifiable to carry out an investigation using the Board's system as it might prove to be of value to patients. I undertook to ensure that I would maintain absolute confidentiality about the prescribing of individual doctors. I adhered to this promise to the NIGHSB right up to the end of my professional life.

With the help of the staff of the pricing bureau I started my first investigation in December 1962. I had decided to examine the prescribing of chloramphenicol. Chloramphenicol is a broad spectrum antibiotic which was a special value in the treatment of typhoid fever but was also effective in many other infectious diseases including whooping cough. It had first been marketed after its discovery, in 1949. In 1951 two American haematologists, Max Wintrobe and Philip Sturgeon, reported that they had each encountered a few patients with aplastic anaemia, which they thought had been caused by damage to the blood forming cells of the bone marrow by chloramphenicol which the patients had received when previously ill with infectious disease.

Evidence from other haematologists in the USA, France and Australia confirmed the suspicion that there was a risk of chloramphenicol occasionally causing severe and sometimes fatal aplastic anaemia and there had been wide publicity about this in the medical press.

I was therefore surprised and worried when my investigation showed that a great deal of chloramphenicol was still being prescribed. In the month of December 1962 there were 3,123 prescriptions for chloramphenicol written by doctors in Northern Ireland, 1,141 for capsules of the drug and 1,982 for a preparation of the antibiotic as a syrup. I and most people that I had consulted including the Chief Medical Officer, Sir George Godber, had assumed that doctors would no longer be prescribing the drug unless it was very specifically indicated, as would have been the case in the treatment of typhoid fever. The fact that so much of the syrup preparation was being prescribed suggested that this antibiotic was still being used for children probably with whooping cough, for which other antibiotics were by then available.

Further analysis brought another interesting fact to light. Of the 756 doctors in general practice at that time, over 500 wrote no prescriptions for chloramphenicol in December 1962, 243 doctors wrote between 1 and 4 prescriptions for the drug during the month and 10 practitioners were responsible for one-quarter of all the prescriptions written.

This first investigation was a hard, time consuming and painstaking task using the Hollerith cards and then tracing back to the original prescriptions written by the doctors. But because the results were so unexpected I felt they had to be independently confirmed and I carried out another similar investigation of the prescribing of chloramphenicol in 1964. In this second investigation the total number of prescriptions written for the drug was smaller, 1,648 prescriptions, but the pattern of prescribing remained the same and interestingly the very high prescribers of the drug in 1962 were still the high prescribers in 1964.

This phenomenon I was later to describe as

'perseveration'. It is not surprising that doctors go on prescribing the medicines they are used to prescribing, rather like the housewife who had her own repertoire of special recipes which she uses repeatedly for her dinner parties.

The introduction of the computer

In 1966 the NIGHSB abandoned the Hollerith cards and began to use a fixed frame computer which was installed by the Northern Ireland government at Stormont Castle and was used for a number of different purposes by government departments. It was also used by the Northern Ireland General Health Services Board for the work of prescription pricing.

This made my work much easier and faster and over the next seven years I and my colleagues, Peter Elmes and Helen Hood produced a whole series of papers showing the great differences in the prescribing habits of doctors, the changes which occurred when new drugs were introduced or when old ones became unpopular and the very interesting differences in drug usage in different parts of Northern Ireland. Amongst the drugs studied were insulin, oral hypoglycaemic drugs, hypnotics, bronchodilators and anti-hypertensive drugs.

Into Europe

In 1969 I was invited to Oslo to take part in a meeting arranged by WHO on 'Drug consumption in Europe'.

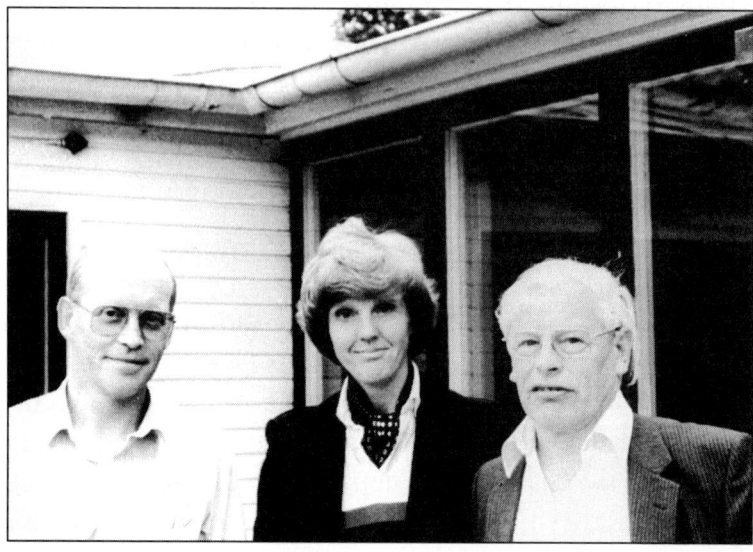

Figure 7.3: Professor Per Lund and Dr Barbro Westerholm, Chief Medical Officer of Sweden, with me in Stockholm.

This meeting was called as a consequence of an investigation of the sales of antibiotic drugs in European countries by Dr Engels, Chief Medical Officer of Sweden and Dr Siderius, a pharmacist in the Dutch Ministry of Health. Their survey, done in 1966–7, had shown great differences in the antibiotics that were used in different countries. For instance in most countries chloramphenicol was little used, but in Germany it constituted 25% of the sales of all antibiotics.

Apart from their data about sales, which they recognised as only a rough measure of drug use, no firm data were presented at that meeting other than those presented by me. My data on drug prescribing in Northern Ireland were received with enormous interest and after I had given my paper Dr Per Lund of Oslo approached me. He told me that he thought he could get similar data to mine in Norway and he proposed that we should collaborate.

I was delighted about this and we started immediately to plan a comparison of the use of drugs in Northern Ireland and Norway. But a few weeks later I received a letter from Dr Barbro Westerholm of Stockholm. She had been at the meeting in Oslo, had heard my paper and in effect said that anything the Norwegians could do the Swedes could do better! Thus started an exciting collaboration which was to result eventually in the creation of a Drug Utilization Research Group, DURG, under the aegis of the World Health Organisation, and in the publication by WHO in 1979 of an extensive report of our work. One of the first of our investigations was into the prescribing of Vitamin B12 which is described in the next chapter.

Conclusion

Let no one doubt how tragic the thalidomide disaster was for the children born with arm or leg deformities and for their parents. But tragic as it was it led to the very necessary development of new and strict legislation in this and other countries to improve the safety of drugs.

It also led to the studies on drug use of which the

first were those I did in Northern Ireland and which within a few years were to be incorporated into the work of the Drug Utilisation Research Group (DURG) of the World Health Organisation.

CHAPTER 8

Vitamin B12

The very name 'pernicious anaemia' recalls for me the great fear that still persisted when I was young in the minds of my parents and their contemporaries of a disease which in the first part of this century had always been fatal. Its victims were usually past middle age, of varied economic status, of either sex and, once the diagnosis had been made, had an expectation of life of between one and three years.

Although it is known as Addison's anaemia, there is some doubt whether the patient described in 1855 by Thomas Addison, physician at Guy's hospital, really had pernicious anaemia. His patient lacked any of the clinical features of which a patient with well established pernicious anaemia might have been expected to have had; a sore mouth, a red glossy tongue, gastritis, slight jaundice and numbness and tingling of the fingers and feet, which might progress to paralysis caused by degeneration of lateral and dorsal columns of the spinal cord with or without visual defects and dementia due to cerebral damage.

The development of good microscopes and the ability to count the red cell content of the blood by using a ruled counting chamber and the introduction of methods of measuring the haemoglobin content of blood had shown by the first quarter of this century, that the commonest form of anaemia was caused by recurrent loss of blood and an iron deficient diet. In this anaemia the red cells are small or microcytic, fewer in number and contain less haemoglobin than the red cells of a healthy person. Malnutrition, menstruation, frequent pregnancies and, in the tropics, malaria were major factors in its world wide distribution. It was and still is a common cause of ill health and debility, but it responds to treatment with iron tablets and better diet.

In contrast, pernicious anaemia was a rare disease. It was a macrocytic anaemia with large and irregular red cells. The anaemia was accompanied by a reduction in the number of white cells and platelets in the circulating blood. The patients's condition deteriorated relentlessly and there was no known remedy.

In the early 1920s some thought pernicious anaemia was primarily a disorder of red cell formation similar perhaps to the leukaemias. Some thought it was caused by a toxin that destroyed red cells. Others suspected it was nutritional, for had not beri-beri and scurvy been recently shown to be due to a lack of Vitamin B or Vitamin C in a patient's diet.

Interest in nutritional causes of anaemia increased in the later 1920s because of the wonderful series of feeding experiments carried out by George Whipple, a physician in Boston, New England. He had developed a system of bleeding dogs every fortnight until the haemoglobin level was 50% of normal. His dogs were then given a 'control' diet of salmon and bread, which contained very little iron, and the amount of blood which had to be taken from the dog at fortnightly intervals to get the haemoglobin level back to 50% was measured as carefully as possible.

Then the dogs were fed other diets. Diets which contained beef, liver, spinach and other protein and iron containing foods. Some of these diets, especially those with a high content of beef or liver, speeded up regeneration of the blood, so that each fortnight much larger amounts of blood had to be taken from the animal if the 50% level of haemoglobin was to be again reached.

Then instead of giving iron containing food he gave iron salts. In Whipple's study giving iron salts did not seem to help blood regeneration. But this perverse finding is I think explained by the fact that the iron preparation he chose to use was Bland's pills which contained ferrous carbonate. These pills were later shown to be a poor source of iron for the pills pass almost unchanged through the gut. But at that time it was thought that it was the iron content of normal foods that was important in treatment.

George Minot

The discovery of insulin at the University of Toronto in 1921–2 was one of the most dramatic events in the history of medicine. One of those whose life was saved just in the nick of time was George Minot. He had developed severe diabetes in 1921 when he was aged

35. Insulin was obtained for him early in 1923 by Elliot Joslin, who was later to be one of the great experts in the treatment of diabetes.

George Minot was an Associate Professor of Medicine at Harvard Medical School. He had a major interest in blood diseases, especially pernicious anaemia, and he was very impressed by Whipple's work. In retrospect he interpreted Whipple's finding wrongly for Whipple's dogs had an iron deficiency anaemia and it was probably the iron content of the diet which was the critical part of their treatment.

Minot started to advise his patients with pernicious anaemia to eat beef and liver. He had noticed that many of them lived on a very limited and selective diet and often expressed a strong dislike of meat – not perhaps surprising if they had troublesome gastritis. His thinking was that there was something in the diet of these patients which was missing and that their anaemia was a form of deficiency disease.

Some of the patients seemed to improve on the diet that he recommended and in 1925 Minot asked William Murphy, a physician at the adjacent Peter Bent Brigham Hospital, to join him in carrying out a rigorous trial of a special diet containing 'an abundance of food rich in complete proteins and iron, particularly liver, and relatively low in fat'.

This special diet contained 120–240 grams of lightly boiled beef liver daily. It was a very unpleasant diet to take. It required enormous patience and persistence to persuade patients to continue to take it. Originally

Minot and Murphy intended to study ten patients, but as the initial results were encouraging this number was increased.

On 4 May 1926 Minot and Murphy reported to a meeting of the Association of American Physicians the consistent improvement in the anaemia of forty-five patients with pernicious anaemia who had received the special diet. The increase in red cell level was always preceded by an increase in the young red cells, the reticulocytes, in the peripheral blood.

So a man whose own life had been saved by the discovery of insulin brought hope and life to patients in whom the diagnosis of pernicious anaemia had up to that time been a death certificate. The impact of the work was enormous and in 1934 its world-wide recognition was confirmed by the award of the Nobel Prize in Physiology and Medicine to Whipple, Minot and Murphy.

Further developments

It was unpleasant to eat a pound of raw liver every day, even if it was life saving. It was assumed that there must be some anti-anaemic factor in liver and not surprisingly great efforts were made to identify and isolate this factor. Very soon a number of liver fractions and liver extracts, which were as effective as the raw liver and more palatable, were available. But it was slow work as the only way to test effectiveness was by seeing if a new preparation would or would not produce an increase in the reticulocyte count in a untreated sufferer of pernicious anaemia.

Then in 1929 a very puzzling and indeed astonishing discovery was made by William Castle working at the Boston City Hospital. How was it, he must have argued, that a normal person did not need to eat a pound of liver a day? Castle knew that some five years previously Dr Hurst at Guy's Hospital had shown that patients with pernicious anaemia had achlorhydria. Hurst had suggested that pernicious anaemia might be secondary to the gastric atrophy which these patients had.

Castle planned an ingenious experiment to throw light on this problem. He fed patients with untreated pernicious anaemia with 200 grams of steak for ten days. As expected, no increase in reticulocyte count was observed.

Then he fed 300 grams of steak to a normal healthy man. An hour later he aspirated the contents of the stomach. Over the next few days portions of this aspirated steak were given by stomach tube to a patient with pernicious anaemia. Within six days a rise in reticulocyte count was observed and then the red cell count started to increase and the anaemia to be corrected.

Gastric juice from a normal person by itself did not produce any increased reticulocyte; there had to be some reaction between normal gastric juice and the steak; Castle's hypothesis was that there was some intrinsic factor in the gastric juice that combined with some extrinsic factor in the steak.

The next year there was another surprising observation. This time it was made by a German physician, Professor Gänsslen. He showed that there was no need for patients to eat liver. A very small dose of a protein free liver extract injected intramuscularly was as potent as a dose 30 to 60 times as large given by mouth.

The identification of the cause of pernicious anaemia

When I was a student in the early 1940s it was still widely accepted that pernicious anaemia was a disease of unknown origin in which there was atrophy of the mucosal lining of the stomach leading to a severe reduction or absence of an 'intrinsic factor' which was needed to allow absorption of an 'external factor' which was present in liver and liver extracts.

Patients could be treated and kept in excellent health either by being given enormous doses of liver or liver extract by mouth or by being given small injections of liver extracts. The injections were the usual method of treatment chosen. The injections had to be given once every three or four weeks and the treatment had to continue throughout the patient's life.

It was not until 1948 that the nature of the 'external factor' was identified. In the Merk laboratories in the USA and a few weeks later quite independently in the Glaxo laboratories in England, it was shown that the 'external factor' was cyancobalamine. It was soon

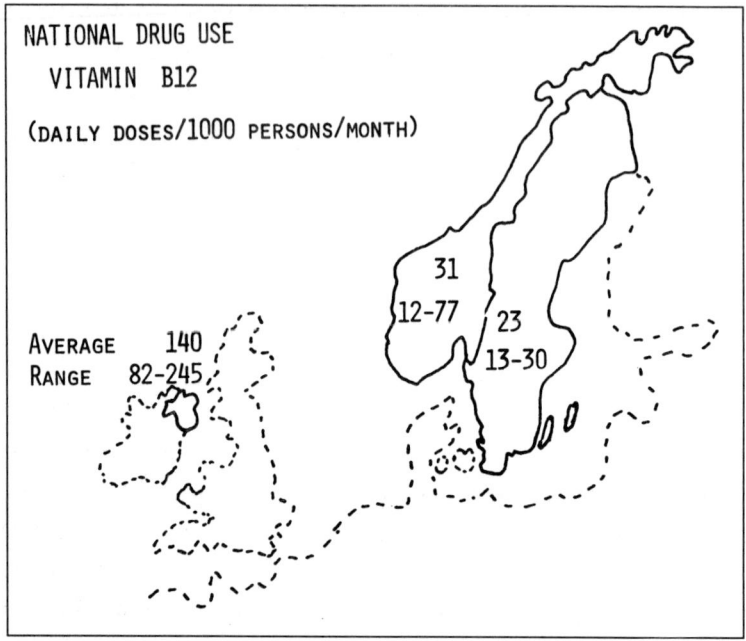

NATIONAL DRUG USE

VITAMIN B12

(DAILY DOSES/1000 PERSONS/MONTH)

AVERAGE   140
RANGE   82-245

31
12-77 / 23
13-30

Figure 8.1: Use of Vitamin B12 in Northern Ireland, Norway and Sweden in 1972. The figures are doses, per thousand of the population, per month.

possible to give small and painless injections of cyan-cobalamine or Vitamin 12 as it was called. These injections had to continue throughout the patient's life.

In 1966 the nature of the 'intrinsic factor' in the gastric juice of healthy people was shown to be a glycoprotein and more recently it has been shown that the absence of this in the patients with pernicious anaemia is caused by damage to the cells of the gastric mucosa by autoimmune antibodies. This incidentally explained why patients with pernicious anaemia were sometimes found to suffer from other autoimmune diseases such as hypothyroidism, thyrotoxicosis, adrenal insufficiency, myasthenia gravis and vitiligo.

Despite these advances in our knowledge, the treatment of pernicious anaemia is still by regular repeated injections of vitamin B12, cyancobalamine or more usually these days, hydroxy-cyancobalamine.

Drug utilization studies

I became interested in the prescribing of Vitamin B12 in 1970. That I did so was a strange and unforseen consequence of the thalidomide tragedy. It is a good example of how in science we so often set out to investigate one problem only to find ourselves exploring some totally unexpected and different problem that has suddenly opened out.

At the beginning of my work on drug prescribing I had became interested in whether the prescribing of drugs by doctors was congruent with the need for drugs.

One of the early investigations that I did in Northern Ireland was on the prescribing of insulin. I felt that no patient who did not need insulin would receive it; on the other hand all diabetics who needed insulin would get it. Use would be congruent with need.

For some time I had been wanting to study the prescribing of Vitamin B12. The hypothesis I wished to test was that the prescribing of Vitamin B12 would not be congruent with need. I believed that the only justifiable reason for prescribing injections of Vitamin

B12 was for patients with pernicious anaemia but I knew that in Northern Ireland it was often prescribed as a 'tonic' for patients who felt out of sorts.

I discussed the problem with colleagues in Norway and Sweden and we agreed that we would look at the prescribing of Vitamin B12 in our three countries.

I remember some weeks later being rung up by Dr Barbro Westerholm from Stockholm. She was anxious to tell me that the use of Vitamin B12 in Sweden was far in excess of the need. She estimated that there were on average 23 patients per 1000 of the population (range 13–30 from region to region) being prescribed Vitamin B12 which she thought was disgracefully high.

I told her that Dr Per Lund had given me the data from Norway. There it was being given on an average of 31 doses per 1000 of the population (range 12–77) per month. Then I told her that in Northern Ireland the prescribing of Vitamin B12 was far higher than in Norway or Sweden. The average was 140 doses per 1000 of the population per month, and that the greatest use was in the rural areas of Counties Tyrone and Fermanagh.

This international comparison of the prescribing Vitamin B12 was the first of many that have since been done which show fascinating differences in prescribing in different countries. It has become clear that the prescribing of drugs, which we had naively assumed to have been done solely on a rational basis, is profoundly influenced by traditions, doctors' concepts of disease, patients' expectations of treatment, the marketing and advertising by drug firms, the misconceptions of the media and the different health service policies in different countries especially policies concerning the reimbursement of the cost of prescription charges.

It is perhaps not surprising that this work on the prescribing of Vitamin B12 played an important part in the birth of a new discipline of drug utilisation studies, which my colleague, Folke Sjoqist of Stockholm has perspicaciously called pharmaco-epidemiology. It was work which changed my life greatly for it was to be fully supported by the World Health Organisation.

Epilogue

A s I prepared these eight chapters for my publisher I gave thought to five issues concerning drugs on which I feel it is appropriate for me to comment briefly.

1. The difficulties in planning medical research

It has been, and always will be, difficult to foresee how some new and unexpected discovery will change our concepts of disease and alter the nature of the research which is thought to be relevant. It is not uncommon for effective treatment to be based on concepts subsequently shown to be wrong. Digitalis was at one time thought to act not on the heart but on the kidney. Dr Minot thought raw liver would be the right treatment for pernicious anaemia because of its iron content.

2. The importance of experimental work on animals

If we can throw light on physiology, pharmacology or pathology by animal experiments, I believe, that as doctors and scientists, we have a duty to do them. Such work has helped us enormously in the past and is still necessary to relieve human suffering. I understand the sentiments of anti-vivisectionists but, too often when I have met them, I have felt that they had little experience of the human suffering caused by disease. Too often their 'crusade' has a strong element of self-gratification. They so clearly felt 'better than others' because they were so dedicated to animals.

3. The ethical problems of research on humans

The planning and execution of research in patients or healthy volunteers demands the highest professional, scientific and ethical qualities of all research workers. The responsibility of such research being done in my Department always weighed heavily on me and my colleagues. But it was always a joy to find how ready patients were to co-operate. I remember being very deeply touched by one lady who told me that she owed her life to research that had been carried out in other patients with leukaemia and that she felt it was her duty to help in the advancement of knowledge that might help others. Many who have benefited from modern medicine, surgery, obstetrics or anaesthesia feel similarly indebted.

4. Risk versus benefit in the use of

There is always a balance between the benefits that may be derived from the use of a drug and any ill effects it may cause, usually infrequently but occasionally so serious, as was the case with thalidomide, that the use of the drug must be discontinued.

It was to make such decisions about drug use that the Committee on Safety of Drugs was created. In my opinion that Committee and its successors have carried out a difficult task with exemplary care.

The British National Formulary is a compact source of information for doctors about the use, effects, doses and possible adverse reactions of all drugs available in this country. A new edition is published every six months by the British Medical Association and the Royal Pharmaceutical Society. It is independent of both the pharmaceutical industry and the Ministry of Health. It has made a major contribution to the quality of prescribing in general practice and the hospital service.

5. The rewards of research

In my experience research is difficult, time consuming and often frustrating. But the satisfaction, indeed sometimes the excitement, of discovering something of help to patients is enormous. The pressure to give service to the sick in our Health Service may at times conflict with the time and effort needed in the search for new knowledge – yet that new knowledge may be of enormous service to countless patients.

Further Reading

For all chapters the reader will find relevant information in *The Pharmacological Basis of Therapeutics*. Goodman, L. S. and Gilman, A. First edition 1941, 2nd edition 1955 and 3rd edition 1965. New York Macmillan.

Chapter 1. Quinine

Duran-Reynolds, M. L. *The Fever Bark Tree*. London, Allen, 1947
Memoranda on Medical Disease in Tropical and Subtropical Areas. London, War Office, HMSO, 1942
Pascol, G. 'Infectious diseases now'. *Quarterly Journal of Medicine* 186 (1993) 233
Shannon, J. A. *Journal of Clinical investigation* (1948), special supplement
Thompson, C. J. S. 'The history and lore of chinchona'. *British Medical Journal* 2 (1928), 1188

Chapter 2. Curare

Bernard, C. *An Introduction to the Study of Experimental Medicine* (1865), translated by H. C. Greene. USA, Schuman, 1949

McIntyre, A. R. *Curare; its History, Nature and Clinical use.* University of Chicago Press, 1947

Chapter 3. Digitalis

Aranson, A. K. *An Account of the Foxglove and its Medical Uses, 1785–1985* (Reprint of William Withering's book (1785) with a commentary on modern work.) Oxford University Press, 1985
Cushney, A. R. *The Action and Uses in Medicine of Digitalis and its Allies.* London, Longman Green, 1925
Lewis, T. *Clinical Disorders of the Heart Beat.* London, Shaw, 1920

Chapter 4. Sulphonamides

Long, P. H. and Bliss, E. A. *The Clinical and Experimental Use of Sulfanilimide, Sulfapyridine and Allied Compounds.* New York, Macmillan, 1939

Chapter 5. Penicillin

Fraser, I. *Blood, Sweat and Cheers.* London, the Memoir Club, Oxford University Press, 1989
Hare, R. *The Birth of Penicillin.* London, Allen & Unwin, 1970

Further Reading

Chapter 6. Streptomycin

Cochrane, A. L. 'Effectiveness and Efficiency'. Nuffield Provincial Hospital Trust, 1972

Daniels, M. and Hill, A. B. 'Chemotherapy of tuberculosis in young adults. An analysis of the combined results of three Medical Research Council trials'. *British Medical Journal* 1 (1952) 1162–68

Hinshaw, H. C. 'Historical note on earliest use of steptomycin in clinical tuberculosis'. *American Review of Tuberculosis* 70 (1954) 9–14

Wakeman, S. A. *The Conquest of Tuberculosis*. London, Cambridge University Press, 1964

Chapter 7. Thalidomide

Wade, O. L. *Adverse Reactions to Drugs*. London, Heinemann, 1970

Wade, O. L. 'The concept of drug utilisation studies'. *Studies of Drug Utilisation*. Copenhagen, European series No. 8, WHO Regional Publications, 1979

Chapter 8. Vitamin B12

Wintrobe, M. M. *Blood Pure and Eloquent. A Story of Discovery, of People and Ideas*. New York, McGraw-Hill, 1980